"Our brains need stories of how other constraints so we might know our own hard too. Julie poignantly offers herself and the us as a reminder that often life's most difficult struggles can also be our most powerful assignments."

—**Katherine Wolf**, survivor, advocate, and
author of *Suffer Strong* and *Hope Heals*

"With incredible transparency and vulnerability, Julie shares the message so many people need to hear who struggle with mental illness, depression, or suicidal thoughts. She not only helps them understand they are not alone, but gives them a glimpse of how precious life is, how much they are loved by God and others, and how He can heal them and use their pain for a purpose. *Joyful Sorrow* is the perfect dose of hope that can not only change lives, but save them."

—**Tracie Miles**, author for Proverbs 31 Ministries; founder of the
Living Unbroken Divorce Recovery Program

"So many books about mental health in the world today tend to be unbalanced. They either use only science to talk about disorders, or minimize struggles and put the responsibility on the person to 'just' pray about it, hinting at mental health being a faith issue. Julie does a wonderful job of explaining how we can use God-given tools like medication and therapy to help sufferers manage symptoms and learn skills for daily life, but she also points out that without the true hope God provides, we are still incomplete. As she writes, 'in the Kingdom of God, the one who embraces their weakness proclaims God's worth through their humility,' Julie speaks in a raw and vulnerable manner in which we can relate. She, like Jesus, uses language we can understand to explain biblical principles, and allows us to see how very much God loves us. She gives the reader a balanced perspective that points them in the right direction for true healing, whether it be on this earth, or in eternity."

—**Heather Annis**, M.S., LPC, The Center
for Christian Counseling and Care

"This is a needed message. A powerful story. *Joyful Sorrow* is a lifeline for anyone struggling with their mental health."

—**Meredith Brock**, Proverbs 31 Ministries, executive director
of strategy and business development

"Julie's story resonated with me in a haunting remembrance of how my own immediate family has been impacted by mental illness, depression, and suicidal thoughts and attempts. It would be easy to be enveloped in the sadness that comes from caring for others who experience a dark night of the soul, but Julie provides her story with hope—a hope found in how Christ provides freedom to the captives. I'm grateful she is sharing her story so others will be encouraged, whether they are personally experiencing the same struggles or ministering to others with compassionate understanding."

—**Kelly King**, manager of magazines/devotional publishing and women's ministry training, Lifeway Christian Resources

"You will want more than one copy of this book! Julie transparently depicts the struggle of mental illness paired with our beautiful hope found in Jesus. She brings to light helpful tools and transformational truth to actively push back darkness."

—**Amy Cordova**, missions and women's ministry partner, Oklahoma Baptists

Julie Busler

JOYFUL
sorrow

Breaking Through the
Darkness of Mental Illness

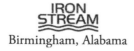

IRON
STREAM
Birmingham, Alabama

Joyful Sorrow

Iron Stream Media
100 Missionary Ridge
Birmingham, AL 35242
IronStreamMedia.com

Copyright © 2022 by Julie Busler

No part of this publication may be reproduced, stored in a retrieval system, or transmitted in any form or by any means—electronic, mechanical, photocopying, recording, or otherwise—without the prior written permission of the publisher.

Iron Stream Media serves its authors as they express their views, which may not express the views of the publisher. While all the stories in this book are true, some of the details and names have been changed or deleted to protect the storyteller's identity.

Library of Congress Control Number: 2022932154

Unless otherwise noted, all Scripture quotations are from THE HOLY BIBLE, NEW INTERNATIONAL VERSION® NIV® Copyright © 1973, 1978, 1984 by International Bible Society® Used by permission. All rights reserved worldwide.

Scripture quotations taken from the Amplified® Bible (AMP), Copyright © 2015 by The Lockman Foundation. Used by permission. www.lockman.org

Scripture quotations marked CSB have been taken from the Christian Standard Bible®, Copyright © 2017 by Holman Bible Publishers. Used by permission. Christian Standard Bible® and CSB® are federally registered trademarks of Holman Bible Publishers.

Scripture quotations marked (ESV) are from The Holy Bible, English Standard Version® (ESV®), copyright © 2001 by Crossway, a publishing ministry of Good News Publishers. Used by permission. All rights reserved.

Scripture quotations marked NASB are taken from the (NASB®) New American Standard Bible®, Copyright © 1960, 1971, 1977, 1995, 2020 by The Lockman Foundation. Used by permission. All rights reserved. www.lockman.org

Scripture quotations marked (NLT) are taken from the Holy Bible, New Living Translation, copyright © 1996, 2004, 2007, 2013, 2015 by Tyndale House Foundation. Used by permission of Tyndale House Publishers, Inc., Carol Stream, Illinois 60188. All rights reserved.

Cover design by twoline || Studio
ISBN: 978-1-56309-558-0 (paperback)
ISBN: 978-1-56309-559-7 (e-book)

1 2 3 4 5—26 25 24 23 22

*To the man who continually reminds me that he chose me, Ryan.
You have shown me Christ's love repeatedly in the way you love me for
better or for worse, and in sickness and in health. You are precious to
me, and I love our life together.*

*To my therapist, Christa. Thank you for the wisdom you share, the
tools you equip me with, and the way you have helped me change my
thinking so that I can live out the lessons in this book. You are an
answer to prayer.*

Contents

Acknowledgments

When I was learning the lessons within these covers, I never anticipated that they would one day become a book. These lessons were learned and journaled in the year following our move home from Turkey during a time where even just getting out of bed was difficult. I knew there was more to the abundant life Jesus speaks of, and in pursuit of that, I began a journey with the Lord through His Word. I felt as though I had been removed from the frontlines of ministry in Turkey and discarded in small town Oklahoma, but little did I know that as I obediently sought Him day in and day out in the quiet morning hours before my children woke up, He was writing a story that would soon move beyond my beat-up leather journal out into the world for all to read. I now see the preciousness of those days where I was tucked away with just Him, abiding, learning, wrestling, growing and eventually thriving. The enemy almost took me out, but to that I say with confidence, "You intended to harm me, but God intended it for good to accomplish what is now being done, the saving of many lives" (Genesis 50:20).

To Jamy Fisher, who sat with me every Thursday as I would share what the Lord was teaching me. You peered into my journal with acceptance of me right where I was, giving me the courage to open up to you rather than isolate. You affirmed what the Lord was teaching me, celebrated the growth, and comforted me on days I couldn't quite comprehend the suffering

I was enduring. Your companionship during the darkest days helped me see Jesus and believe His promises. Every life that is touched by this book is an extension of your ministry to me. I love you.

To my children, Boston, Evangeline, Clementine, and Abel, who have experienced their own hard days as I fought for life, particularly during hospital stays. You four are among God's sweetest gifts to me and this great calling of mothering you is not lost on me. Thank you for loving me, believing in me, and championing everything I do. It is an absolute joy when you tell me how you shared Jesus with a friend at school by sharing my story. It's our story, dear ones, and may He receive all the glory.

Necoe Bandy and Erin Allred, my loyal friends, who have loved me during every season. The way you have encouraged me to write and have celebrated each milestone along the way has been essential to this book getting out into the world. Even when my faith has faltered, you have always been quick to remind me that I am here for such a time as this. Thank you for praying for me faithfully and reminding me often just how loved I am. Kelli Ann Rollins, I am also so grateful for you. It remains fresh in my mind the many times you have prayed over me and supported me in this journey. Your delight in God's Word is contagious.

Amy Cordova, thank you for believing in me. From the moment I met you, you have been a voice of encouragement and wisdom, as well as one of my dear friends. Thank you for the opportunities you've given me to serve our state alongside you, and for giving me various platforms to share my message of hope from. I remember sitting with you at lunch in Shawnee and timidly admitting to you that I think I wanted to write a book. You celebrated this dream with me, but also reminded me to keep doing the next right thing. You've helped me focus on just the daily task of loving God and loving others. Little did I know that my book was being written out of the overflow of doing those things.

Sandy Wisdom-Martin, thank you from the bottom of my heart for guiding me and helping bring this book out into the world. I will never forget getting the phone call from you, asking me what I thought about Iron Stream Media publishing my book. It's an honor to serve alongside you with the WMU, and I hope you know what I tremendous gift your support has been to me.

Tracie Miles, you have been an invaluable part of this book becoming a reality. It was an honor to be mentored by you, for without your guidance, I never would have known where to begin writing. Thank you for believing in my message and for the way you have helped me navigate the publishing world. I am forever grateful for you.

To my home church, Immanuel Baptist Church, thank you for supporting me and allowing me to share my story at our women's event in 2020. Very few knew my story and I was mortified to share any of it publicly. You, however, embraced my story when I finally felt led to share it. From that women's event, an entire ministry has grown as well as this book. You were a safe place to first share, giving me confidence to continue sharing.

To the gracious people of Iron Stream Media—I can never express the depth of my gratitude for the way you have believed in my message and brought it to the printed page.

And finally, my dear Ryan, being your wife is the greatest honor of my life. You have taken care of me, advocated for me, fought for me, and I am here today because of you. Living in Turkey was your dream, and the way you laid it down for my sake, is a picture of Christ's sacrificial love for His bride. Here's to our bright future together—may He continue to show us where He is working and let us be a part of it. I love you.

Introduction

My mind was made up. Having already contemplated details, I was waiting for the right moment to end my life at only thirty-four years of age. I was a wife, mother, and follower of Jesus who lived to make Him known in the predominately Muslim country of Turkey, and yet the very hope I proclaimed somehow slipped through my fingers.

What's frightening is that no one knew. How can a Christian struggle with such darkness? I honestly didn't know. I was ashamed, so I didn't tell.

For years, intrusive thoughts were a hidden plague within my mind, beginning after I witnessed the graphic death of my mother when I was a teenager. Her death was beyond my ability to cope. It was traumatic.

My teen years were supposed to be that carefree season in life I would look back on as the good ole days, but my mother's cancer gave me a different narrative. Several years later, my thoughts only grew more disturbing after my dad's death by suicide shattered what was left of my life.

What began as thoughts of despair slowly blossomed into life-threatening commands that painted death in my broken brain as glamorous, even courageous. I was in pain and death would remedy that. My thinking possessed a great paradox.

My faith was in Christ and my hope was in a secured future with Him. But my coexisting irrational, albeit logical, suicidal thinking pulled my faith-filled gaze away from Jesus and focused solely on the temporary pain that I believed was unendurable. This double-mind created instability. I supposed I was suffering from depression and Post-traumatic Stress Disorder (PTSD), but the isolating, vicious cycle of hiding everything with unfortunate ease behind a smiling, friendly exterior was the only way I knew to survive.

The undiagnosed, untreated mental illness I was living with was killing me, and no one, not even my husband, suspected what I was contemplating. Depression trapped me like an excruciating night terror that seemed impossible to wake up from. When my children were at school and my husband was at work, the paralyzing darkness would often strap me to the bed in hopeless defeat. Tyrannical thoughts, graphic images, and imaginings consumed my mind, nearly causing irrevocable action on my part.

What I now understand to be illness highjacked my thinking, leading me to believe with irrational certainty that I was a burden on my family. Thoughts of living the rest of my life without relief were an insurmountable obstacle that led to my secret obsession with suicide. There was only one missing thing: the note. With the assumption that it would be found after I was gone, I hid away in a small room in our apartment in Istanbul, Turkey. I slid down the wall and sat on the cold tile floor while my children played in the other room. I opened up the notepad on my phone and typed this simple goodbye: "I guess I'm just like my dad. I'm sorry."

Details of my dad's suicide surged through my mind at lightning speed with each letter I typed. While seven years crept by since he left me orphaned with his one pull of the trigger, my heart was still as raw as the moment I read his own suicide note.

God would eventually use my father's death to create compassion in me for those who are dying without hope. Yet, even after seeing how good could miraculously come from such tragedy, the palpable pain created a desperate appetite in my inner being to make it stop. Devastating circumstances can confuse a mind that once grasped truth. Suffering fed my deep feelings of loneliness despite being surrounded by my loving family. As angry as I was at my dad, somewhere along the way I started identifying with my earthly father over my Heavenly Father.

Despite not wanting to be like him, I started to believe that being like him was inevitable. As a mother, part of me wouldn't wish that uniquely devastating pain upon my children, but I was also an abandoned daughter left behind by her dad's choice. I was caught between two different perspectives, but the pain I felt as a daughter started to overshadow the strength I possessed as a mother. Shame created a cavern between my heart and the Lord. God never left me, but I unknowingly pushed Him away without even realizing it was happening. Despair ensued, enforcing the lie that my only choice was to follow my dad's footsteps in leaving a legacy of loss.

I continued sitting on that cold floor in Istanbul, clutching my phone as I tried to make sense of how I inched closer and closer to making what I see now as the biggest mistake of my life. As a lover of words, I envisioned a more eloquent goodbye. Unfortunately, even as a child of Light, sickness and sin wrapped my mind in such darkness that even my creativity was held captive. The writer in me couldn't muster up anything beyond those two short sentences. I needed help, and although help would come, "Darkness is my closest friend" (Psalm 88:18) became my story and my song.

I glanced at the words on my phone and thought "How pathetic." With a sigh of defeat, I erased the note. My cheeks flushed with shame while the father of all lies whispered "failure" over me. I walked out of that room and interacted with my family completely disregarding what took place just minutes prior. My capacity to understand the devastation I was close to inflicting on them was nonexistent. I was sick. I needed hope. And the enemy was using all of this to his advantage.

It wouldn't be until months later after receiving help and relocating back to the United States that I would really ponder that short, sad note I nearly left behind. As I went over every word thoughtfully in my mind, while sitting alone on our porch in small town Oklahoma, this phrase interrupted my thoughts:

"I could either write a short note of despair or a whole book of hope."

I have chosen the latter. A book of hope, pointing to Jesus, our one and only hope, is exactly what I pray this book will be. Learning to thrive in the midst of depression has been a long journey with imperfect progress along the way. Who am I to address the multifaceted, often misunderstood, topic of mental illness Christians tend to experience in isolated shame? I am neither a doctor nor a therapist, but I am a follower of Christ who is deeply acquainted with depression as well as with Scripture.

To those who are struggling to find help and hope, the Lord has led me to write the resource I wish was available to me in the days of crisis that nearly ended in death. These pages contain the lessons that saved my life, and it's an honor to share them with you.

The apostle Paul's words to the Corinthians, "sorrowful, yet always rejoicing" (2 Corinthians 6:10) have come to be my resting place as a woman of faith who lives with mental illness. There will always be sorrow over the pain that accompanies depression, but I've learned that the joy of the Lord really can be my strength as I endure. The Lord has enlightened the eyes of my heart, so I understand the hope I am called to as His daughter.

If you are reading this book from a place of despair, hold fast. There is hope which we will look for together. Jesus is the Light, and "the light shines in the darkness, and the darkness has not overcome it" (John 1:5).

1

Healing Starts with Humility

We knew we would live a more isolated life as foreigners in Turkey, but gladly resigned the comfort of community when we picked up our cross and followed Christ to the faraway lands of Central Asia. Loneliness was an ongoing trial for me particularly, but my ache for loved ones back home was interrupted when my mother-in-law visited us in Istanbul in the summer of 2018. As she opened up her suitcase, there were gifts for the kids surrounded by American snacks that you long for overseas, but probably rarely desire stateside. We were excited to show her the unique life we lived as foreigners and even planned on playing tourist alongside her while she visited.

While cognitively I knew I should feel the warmth of joy as I watched my children joyfully swarm their grandma, I felt a hollow disconnect. Past trauma continued to infiltrate my present reality, leaving me continually going through the motions of life while feeling numb internally. In the middle of her visit, one moment has remained seared in my mind as the beginning of the end of life as we knew it. We were hanging out as a family, soaking in her company, when a thought popped in my mind: While my mother-in-law is here, it would be a great time to kill myself because she could help my husband get the kids home to the US . . . and my body.

In true intrusive thought fashion, that idea was disturbing and arrived unannounced. Although I call the thought disturbing now, at the time I found comfort in this plan that would end my unrelenting pain. That thought was an invader to the beautiful moments happening with my family, and rather than taking it captive and making it obedient to Christ (2 Corinthians 10:5), it captivated me. I continued interacting with my family while harrowing thoughts hidden in the confines of my mind contradicted the plastic smile on my face. How could I, a devoted wife and mother, as well as a child of God, serve my family while silently savoring the evil plans in my mind? How could I hug one of my precious children, and not rationally see what carrying out that plan would do to them?

Maybe you get it.

If you do, then you know what it's like to struggle alone in the dark.

If this is all hitting a little too close to home, just know that I understand. You have thoughts no one would believe. You know the Bible well and continue to study it. You are active in church and well-respected in your community.

But you think about dying. Some days, you long for it. You feel like a burden on your friends and family. And despite knowing Jesus is your hope, a powerful pull toward death. Perhaps the outpouring of Job's heart resonates with you who long for a death that never seems to come.

"Why is light given to those in misery, and life to the bitter of soul, to those who long for death that does not come, who search for it more than for hidden treasure, who are filled with gladness and rejoice when they reach the grave? Why is life given to a man whose way is hidden, whom God has hedged in? For sighing has become my daily food; my groans pour out like water. What I feared has come upon me; what I dreaded has happened to me. I have no peace, no quietness; I have no rest, but only turmoil" (Job 3:20–26).

You feel like you must be crazy. You question your salvation. You also justify away needing help, with shame always close by to keep you isolated. You forgo getting help for a myriad of reasons, one being that you assume you'd never actually follow through with the suicidal thoughts that have infiltrated your mind. You've also convinced yourself that Christians shouldn't struggle in this way, leading to your silent suffering as a way to mask the inner turmoil.

Vocational ministry might even further complicate your feelings. But that prideful mindset is dangerous as many lovers of Jesus have lost their battle with despair. No station or vocation in life is immune to suicide.

Suicidal thoughts can accompany many conditions such as depression, anxiety, PTSD, and bipolar disorder. "Approximately one-third of individuals with bipolar II disorder report a lifetime history of suicide attempt,"[1] and "approximately 5%–6% of individuals with schizophrenia die by suicide, about 20% attempt suicide on one or more occasions, and many more have significant suicidal ideation."[2] In depressive disorders,

> Thoughts of death, suicidal ideation, or suicide attempts are common. They may range from a passive wish not to awaken in the morning or a belief that others would be better off if the individual were dead, to transient but recurrent thoughts of committing suicide, to a specific suicide plan. More severely suicidal individuals may have put their affairs in order (for example, updated wills, settled debts), acquired needed materials (for example, a rope or a gun), and chosen a location and time to accomplish the suicide. Motivations for suicide may include a desire to give up in the face of perceived insurmountable obstacles, an intense wish to end what

is perceived as an unending and excruciatingly painful emotional state, an inability to foresee any enjoyment in life, or the wish to not be a burden to others.[3]

Because Christians can most certainly struggle with mental illness just like any other human in all of history, it is absolutely possible to struggle with thoughts of dying as a born-again follower of Christ, or even carry out the act. In case no one has ever told you, you are not alone in feeling these things. You live in a fallen body and you have an enemy that wants to convince you that no other Christian would dare dream of death like you do. He's the father of all lies who is relentless and masterful in his mission to murder you. But don't worry, we don't have to fall victim to his schemes. "No, in all these things we are more than conquerors through him who loved us" (Romans 8:37 CSB). You were meant for so much more than simply surviving every dreaded moment you're alive.

You were made for joy.

Joy, however, seemed impossible while I sat silently in front of my family fantasizing about my death. The thought did shock me a little, but the sense of power and accomplishment that it also gave me seemed to shout over the still small voice in me that whispered "*flee.*"

I was not helpless in my moment of temptation despite the magnetic pull I felt toward the sin of suicide. The Bible tells us "No temptation has overtaken you that is not common to man. God is faithful, and he will not let you be tempted beyond your ability, but with the temptation he will also provide the way of escape, that you may be able to endure it. Therefore, my beloved, flee from idolatry" (1 Corinthians 10:13–14 ESV).

That small reminder to flee from the thoughts that tempted me came from the Holy Spirit. Those thoughts weren't just fleeting, they were all-encompassing. They were an idol— something I spent time thinking about, loving, and essentially worshiping. Unfortunately the strong emotions connected to those thoughts that I felt took precedence over the logic and faith I possessed.

While the Spirit was faithful, I was not. But that's who God is, for "If we are unfaithful, he remains faithful, for he cannot deny who he is" (2 Timothy 2:13 NLT).

My rebellion against the Spirit's invitation to obediently flee ended up nearly costing me my life. It was as though the courage I needed to turn years of suicidal ideation into the actual execution of my life was something I finally mustered up. Years of becoming desensitized to dark thoughts snowballed into them pushing the boundary of what was OK in my mind. The desire within me for death eventually grew stronger than my desire to obey Jesus.

It wasn't a willful disobedience, but rather an apathetic drift away from obedience. Depression poisoned my ability to passionately pursue Jesus even though I wanted to. At times I could nurture my relationship with Him despite the dark emotions pulsating through my being, but that ability was slipping through my fingers. My pride paraded around in silence as I sat there convinced I needed to have it all together on the outside for my family. My pursuit of outward perfection left me with a dreadfully neglected inner life. I didn't grasp at the time, however, just how much my struggles were laid bare before the God Who Sees.

The comfort of the thought was found in finally seeing an end in sight to the unrelenting pain that filled each fiber of my being. What I failed to fully comprehend at the time was that when my thoughts crossed the very dangerous threshold from wishful thinking to plans, it was an emergency. I desperately needed professional help, for without intervention it would only be a matter of time before my plans birthed irreversible action. In Proverbs 23:7 (NASB), we learn that as a man "thinks within himself, so he is," and my life was beginning to bear the spoiled fruit of the poisonous thoughts that held my mind captive. I was becoming what I was thinking.

My mind was so enslaved to thoughts of death that I was unable to rationally see how my horrific death would shatter the hearts of those who loved me. I was in severe emotional pain that blinded me from reality. I was sick.

"Your husband loves you," you might say, and although he is a wonderful and lovingly devoted husband, I failed to grasp my worth to him. Mental illness convinced me I was a burden on him rather than his beloved bride whom he cherished.

"Just pray more or have more faith," you might say, but is that what you would say to someone with diabetes or cancer? My suspicion is that you would encourage them to accept the medical help available to them. The same goes for illness in the mind. Yes, prayer and faith have been essential in finding joy, but at that time, my brain was sick and in need of a doctor. This is why they call it mental illness. The world I saw was skewed. It wasn't that I was selfish, it was that I didn't understand the degree of destruction my death would leave behind.

I was convinced I was a burden.

I felt helpless.

I believed the emotional pain I felt would literally kill me.

I was so entangled in sin that a purposeful life was something I no longer cared to pursue.

I was obsessed with worrying how I'd survive all the years of life I assumed were ahead of me. Always and never are two words that became a deadly trap in my thinking. Therapy eventually helped me unearth the toxicity in those absolutes, as well as show me the deadly trap they were in my thinking. Through counseling, I eventually learned that always and never are not just words, but two very powerful mindsets that threaten the hope I am told to hold fast to in Scripture.

"It's always going to be this dark."

"I'm never going to get any better."

Always and never are the absolutes that lose sight of eternity as our feelings blind our knowledge. There is a day unbeknownst to us that the imperfect will pass away as the perfect will be ushered in for all eternity. This is good news that challenges always and never. Jesus is our hope. As a Christian, whose eternity is secured through Christ, this earth is the only hell you will ever know. Your pain has an expiration date. Your mental struggles will cease to exist.

When we entertain always and never, we set the stage for the enemy to present his tired scheme of suicide. A mind that becomes convinced the pain will never end is a mind that sees this irrational plan as the logical means to an end. When your traumatized mind tells you, "This will last forever," pause and remind yourself that given your pain, this is a very typical thought. And this is precisely why getting professional help is such a beautiful thing. Therapy can help teach faulty thought patterns that might otherwise go unnoticed. Once a toxic thought pattern has been recognized, applying the Word of God comes next. Looking at the thoughts that batter your brain through the eyes of Scripture will lead to hope in a way that therapy alone is found wanting.

Once a thought pattern is understood through therapy and held up against what God says, comes the all-important habit of preaching truth yourself. Through Christ, the pain you feel won't last forever. The same power that raised Jesus from the dead lives in you and can resurrect your thoughts. The very act of enduring these thoughts will shape your character and strengthen your hope. And that hope will then, in turn, continue to fight always and never.

It's taken me years to come to this place though. Before I could understand with such clarity, I was single-minded in my pursuit of relief and, unfortunately, I lost the capacity to rationally understand the lies attached to every thought. I wasn't a coward who wanted to give up, but rather I was convinced that leaving this life was the courageous choice that would relieve my family.

All lies. Straight from hell. But lies that even a Christian can believe. And, unfortunately, we do.

That little voice in me wondered if something wasn't quite right with the thoughts I was having, spoke up louder once my mother-in-law flew back to Oklahoma. Upon her arrival to the US, she posted about me on social media. She wrote:

> The thing I have been most impressed with this trip is my beautiful daughter-in-love. She has blown me away with her growth and walk with God and the sweetness she uses in raising my grandchildren. Ryan and Julie make a great team doing life. Julie has embraced the crazy lack of ingredients for just the simplest recipes. She is a master in the kitchen. She has researched and taught herself so much. She is love, real love for her family. She has always blessed me and allowed me to be a mom figure of a sort for her. I am amazed at her creativity and reasoning skills. Her home is a home she has put together with love and constant hard work. She seldom sits still and her children and home show that. She spends time reading the word and growing spiritually to be the woman she was creative to be. My son loves and honors his wife, and my Julie loves and honors him. No mother could be more proud of this family. We can all learn from them.

I mulled over her kind words and was astonished at how I was perceived by the outside world. Despite understanding something wasn't quite right, not knowing how to get help paralyzed me. Honestly, even as a mature Christian who could recite Scripture, I did not know where I stood on mental illness. Was it a faith problem? Was it an illness? Did I just not pray enough or act good enough or have enough willpower?

The questions were an obstacle too large for me to entertain for very long before I'd just shove them all back down again and try to ignore them. But left unattended, they caused such mental disorder that I couldn't understand that even with unanswered questions, it was possible to seek help. It finally did make sense to me, however, that the world perceived me very differently than I truly was.

This realization was crucial. I was trapped in this vicious cycle of living one inner reality encased in a completely alternate reality for the world to see. I didn't want to live this double life; I just didn't know how else to survive. By putting on the happy face and going through the motions, I was surviving, and when there is so much cognitive dissonance, survival is all you're worried about. According to Merriam-Webster dictionary, *cognitive dissonance* is defined as a "psychological conflict resulting from incongruous beliefs and attitudes held simultaneously."

Cognitive dissonance can be distressing. Feelings of guilt, shame, or regret regarding something you've done and therefore hiding it from others is an example of this. So is trying to rationalize a decision you have made or some action you've taken.

For a Christian who strives to live a holy life that shares hope in Christ with others, dealing with suicidal thoughts, planning her death, or even just feeling hopeless, can certainly cause not only distressing dissonance, but feelings of hypocrisy. When your thoughts do not match your behavior or impulses, shame swoops in and silences you from ever telling your secret struggles, and this is precisely where satan wants you.

Struggling, ashamed, isolated, and silent.

Shame's paralysis is no match for the Spirit's power, but there is definitely a struggle between the flesh and spirit found in all Christians. Living in the tension of knowing what is right and wanting to do what is right, but continuing to do what is wrong, is actually the reality of every single believer on this planet. The apostle Paul explained this tension in the book of Romans when he wrote: "For I know that nothing good lives in me, that is, in my flesh. For the desire to do what is good is with me, but there is no ability to do it" (Romans 7:18 CSB). Paul was right. I could not do it on my own despite my desperate attempts.

Suicidal thoughts were not new to me. When my mother died while I was a teenager, watching her life end traumatized me and made death a reality to my naive mind. Prior to her death, I hadn't given dying much thought. But as I watched her writhe in pain, panting until she grew still, trauma changed the nature of my thoughts forever. It was after her death that depression and Post-traumatic Stress Disorder, although undiagnosed and untreated, became the filter through which I experienced the world.

The dangerous thoughts were so mild in the beginning that I didn't even really take notice of them. Thoughts like "I'm so sad," or "How will I survive this pain?" quickly became normal in my daily thinking. Over the years, I seemingly became desensitized to the thoughts.

They were familiar old friends that somehow felt comforting, even slipping by subconsciously. The intrusive thoughts became a constant soundtrack playing in the background of my life. They were the core of who I was. Their increase in severity was so gradual that they grew to a life-threatening danger completely unsupervised. It would just take one slight trigger and my mind would spiral out of control. Despite appearing happy and engaged on the outside, I would feel disconnected from those around me, while a movie reel of trauma would vividly play in my mind. This unauthentic existence was accompanied by shame, despair, a feeling of being trapped, culminating in a desperation for death. A tremendous amount of effort it required for someone who has been traumatized to carry the memories of horror and feelings of complete weakness and helplessness with them, while continuing to function.

I was functioning, but not in the healthy way God desires. In the happy moments, thoughts of suicide were still there. While on adventurous vacations, the feelings of despair were still there. As I delighted in my family, the thoughts of wanting to give up were still strong and steady. You see, they were always there, always tempting, always poisoning me from the inside out while the enemy waited until I snapped.

Shortly after my mother-in-law's trip to Turkey, I knew my life depended on something changing. I told my husband just enough about my struggles for him to realize I needed professional help. He made an appointment for me to be seen by a Turkish psychiatrist and I reluctantly agreed to go.

I will never forget walking through the glass door into the psychiatrist office. Wrought with worry, I felt a cloud of shame cover me completely. And wondered: How will I share Jesus with the Muslim psychiatrist if I am honest with her? Won't my struggles completely invalidate anything I can say about the sufficiency of Christ?

The receptionist handed me a clipboard with a stack of papers to fill out before I could be seen by the doctor. I looked down and read the first question: "Do you feel worthless?"

This popped into my mind first: Well, the right answer (the Jesus answer) is of course not. Of course, I felt worthless and I didn't know how I would ever feel any differently. Any good church girl would put no, but I knew that if I continued to hide behind "right" answers, I might not survive. I circled "yes" and continued down the list, honestly answering the questions no matter what the Bible says is right.

I turned in my paperwork and looked around at the other women in the waiting room. Their heads were bowed, and their eyes focused on the ground radiated sadness.

And then it hit me: I'm just as broken as they are. I finally saw myself on the same playing field as the women who initially inspired my move to Turkey. People who are all broken and in need of a Savior. I saw myself in a more accurate light which was both absolutely necessary in me grasping my great need for help, and sanctifying as I realized my place in relation to the Almighty.

When the doctor eventually called me back, her impeccable English and kindness whisked my worries away. Despite our cultural and religious differences, I found myself opening up to her easily. Although surprised, I began to come to terms with the science of what I was dealing with at this moment when I realized our differences did not hinder her from helping me.

Yes, there was an entire spiritual side of me that needed help, but the physical side of me was finally being treated. She diagnosed me with Major Depressive Disorder and Post-traumatic Stress Disorder, prescribed medication, and scheduled follow-up appointments. Although apprehensive, I started taking the medication out of desperation.

Instead of getting better, I actually grew worse. It would take a long time for doctors to discover an effective combination of medication for me. Suicidal thoughts saturated my mind more than ever—in my dreams, my thoughts, my journal, my Google searches. My body started reacting to the thoughts. I felt an urge to carry them out so strong that I feared I would succumb to their commands. It was the overwhelming temptation you feel when you are on a diet and all you want is dessert. Although I wouldn't have understood it this way at the time, suicidal thoughts were what my mind was worshiping.

They were acting as my god and were summoning me to obey.

After several appointments with my new psychiatrist, I remember sitting in front her while my husband praised my strength. The doctor quickly popped the bubble of perfection I hid inside of when she said to my husband, "Her strength is what makes her so dangerous. People like her basically make themselves be strong and neglect their insides."

I hated her words and rejected their validity, but I have come to understand over time that, yes, a neglected inner life, encased in a meticulously polished shell, leaves a hollowness that is not God's plan for your life.

If you have been raised to believe that showing weakness equates failure, let me tell you that in the kingdom of God, the one who embraces their weakness proclaims God's worth through their humility. Don't hide your weakness; please don't waste it.

Trust in God's allowance of mental illness as a trial that chisels and beautifully shapes you for your good and His glory. With humility comes wisdom. Through Christ, the miraculous can happen—a mentally ill mind can also be a sound mind.

I've learned that my mind with depression and PTSD can also grasp Scripture, pursue holiness, have wisdom, and a flourishing relationship with Jesus. And yes, the medical world has helped me immensely, but only I can choose to follow the Holy Spirit's prompting to boast in my weakness and humbly depend on God, because with "the humble [the teachable who have been chiseled by trial and who have learned to walk humbly with God] there is wisdom and soundness of mind" (Proverbs 11:2 AMP).

Several weeks into receiving care with my Turkish psychiatrist, I remember one appointment in particular where I went into detail with her about the darkness of my thoughts. She nonchalantly paused and told me to go sit in the waiting room so she could talk to my husband for a minute. I obliged, not having any idea how her conversation with him would change the course of my life forever. She called him in and asked him how I was doing.

"Good," he said.

"Actually, she's not," my psychiatrist said in a serious tone. "She is doing worse and needs to be hospitalized immediately."

My husband didn't believe her because I was doing so well on the outside. But that's the thing about suicide—it often shocks the survivors left behind.

The doctor called me back in and instructed me to tell Ryan everything. My coping skills were nonexistent at this point and pretending to be OK was no longer an option. It was gut-wrenching to verbalize his worst nightmare to him. His face bore the shock of my words and I can only imagine the helplessness he felt while his bride confessed her irrational thoughts and plans. My world was crumbling, but his was too.

We must, especially within the Church, come to terms with the reality that a person with depression doesn't always appear sad. Mental illness can often be invisible. The one struggling might be bubbly, accomplished, and concerned about their appearance. There is this filter applied so no one can see the inner chaos that silently suffocates them under the weight of despair.

For this type of person, admitting they need help can seem like an overwhelming obstacle. You don't want to be more of a burden than you already feel that you are. You don't want to ruin your kids' view of you as a good parent. You fear a mental illness diagnosis equals a death to your ministry, and you're scared that if you tell what is really going on inside, people will be disappointed. Your high functionality creates confusion as to whether or not you really need intervention.

Pride sneaks in as a masked intruder, hiding in the shadows while subtly poisoning everything inside of you. Pride is the sin that will most likely blind you from your need for a Savior, but it's difficult to detect this is happening when you're the one diseased by it. It takes root and distorts reality. In the case of mental illness, pride not only kept me from seeking help that would destroy my carefully curated appearance, but it also convinced me that I was too strong to succumb to the illness that was killing me. Proverbs 29:23 (NLT) says, "Pride ends in humiliation, while humility brings honor."

Had I continued to flounder and slowly drown by choice in the sea of life-threatening despair, humiliation would have been my legacy, not honor. There is nothing honorable about suicide. Nothing. What's honorable is asking for help, which I mentioned before takes humility.

At the time I wasn't choosing humility, but rather being allowed to feel the pain of humiliation. The humiliation of needing psychiatric help broke me, but it was in the breaking that I would eventually be put back together by the One who makes things whole.

It wasn't until my meager coping skills ran out that I would finally understand my need for Christ. I was at the end of myself, and by the grace of God, a doctor was provided for me who could see past my mask. God's plan for my healing was in motion, and while there was more difficulty to come, I can look back and confidently say that He never left my side.

My husband, Ryan, never left my side, either, until he was forced to. Before going to the hospital, we went home so I could pack. My husband was numb. He was angry, felt betrayed, was embarrassed, and scared.

I felt more than ever that I was a burden on him and that he would be better off without me. When I asked Ryan about this moment, he remembers it this way: "It didn't seem real. How could my Christian wife who loved to share about Jesus be suicidal? I just sat in the living room while she packed her bags. It was like she was going on a vacation."

Ryan took me to the hospital where we waited together in the lobby, mostly in awkward silence. After thirteen years of marriage, he was reeling, wondering if all those happy years were merely an illusion.

I felt panicked, wanting desperately to comfort him, but not having any words to help him understand. We were in ministry. How on earth would we explain everything we were going through to those who supported us?

While zoned out entertaining anxious thoughts I had no ability to sort out, two Turkish nurses came to admit me. Each took one of my arms and I remember feeling as if I were a prisoner being taken away. Glancing over my shoulder, I saw my husband's worried face that still haunts me to this day. The nurses joined me in a small room for an extensive search that not only stole my dignity but created a frantic desperation to escape deep within.

I was given red rubber shoes and taken to a locked floor of a Turkish psychiatric hospital where I would be cut off from the outside world for several weeks. It wasn't many years prior that I was a housewife in Oklahoma who spent her days cleaning the house, taking care of kids, cooking dinner, and occasionally making a Target run. Being locked away in a foreign mental hospital is something I never could have imagined would be my life.

The hospital staff didn't let my husband come say goodbye to me after being admitted because an all-out breakdown on my part had taken place. When my husband finally persuaded them to let him say goodbye to me, we were given a few moments together. He said, "When she came in the room she was like a caged animal. I gave her a hug and took her wedding ring home."

Being admitted into the hospital was a defining moment in my life. The type of moment that splits your life in two—before and after. As an ax on wood, the split was sudden and not without some rough edges, but in the split would come sanctification.

The hardship is the pathway to holiness. The humility is that pathway to honor.

Each moment of being in the hospital was difficult. Being locked away and alone was hard in and of itself, but having tests and treatments performed on me without my consent left me feeling violated and frightened. It's not that their methods were wrong, it's that I was a foreigner who was stretched to the max beyond my comfort zone in every way thinkable. They performed multiple sessions of electroconvulsive therapy on my brain. While effective, it was extremely disorienting to experience short-term memory loss and have no idea why I was in the hospital after I would wake from each session. "Electroconvulsive therapy (ECT) is a medical treatment most commonly used in patients with severe major depression or bipolar disorder that has not responded to other treatments. ECT involves a brief electrical stimulation of the brain while the patient is under anesthesia."[4]

What made the entire situation unfathomable is that my life had morphed from one that felt as though divine purpose filled every step I took, to one where I was separated from my children being poked and prodded in a Turkish mental hospital.

A number of thoughts ran through my mind often. How did I end up locked away with the very people I came to share hope with? What would people back home in America think of me? Why would God let me have a mental breakdown after six years overseas had equipped us in ministering and loving others more intentionally than ever before?

Proclaiming Christ in the streets of Central Asia had been replaced with being concealed in a hospital that was everything but familiar. My roommate's Quran sat on a table in our room as she would perform her prayers on her prayer rug near my bed. I, however, was denied a Bible no matter how many times I begged. And while Scripture wasn't really on my mind at that time, even if I wanted to find comfort in the Bible, it was forbidden.

For the first time in my life, I was without access to God's Word, and at one point another patient held me down and tried to forcibly convert me to Islam. I was ultimately sedated in order to create peace.

What I now see is that God allowing my mental breakdown was an act of mercy that would ultimately lead to my freedom.

Brokenness often proceeds walking in wholeness. I also started to see that God loves Muslim people, but He also loves ordinary housewives who live with mental illness.

Our mission overseas had been placed on a pedestal above my personal mental health because I placed a certain people group above my importance. But God simply loves. He cared too much about me as His daughter to allow me to pretend any longer.

And so, eventually we were moved back to Oklahoma for me to find the help I needed, but that move was not without trauma. To have your life as you know it suddenly ripped away from you and be relocated to your home country that now feels like a foreign land is disturbing to go through. While doctors finally stabilized me in the Turkish hospital that was my home for several weeks, I was still in a desperately dark place.

2

Feasting in the Valley

I sat nervously in a plastic chair that was said to be weighted so patients couldn't throw it in a fit of rage. Shivering, I glanced around the cold room. I remember being taken aback by how the barrenness of my heart reflected the sterile scene my eyes struggled to make sense of. Men and women from all walks of life sat around me with one thing in common: brokenness. Me, a woman in ministry, sat next to a man on meth. I saw afresh that mental illness is incapable of discrimination.

Upon discharge from the Turkish hospital, we relocated to the United States. Life was a whirlwind and I felt like I was drowning. Still attempting to wrap my head around my recent hospitalization in Turkey, I was also caring for four children, one being a baby. I was exhausted and jetlagged and after a failed attempt to take my life, I was placed in a psychiatric hospital in Oklahoma. This was my second hospitalization in a month.

The deadness I felt inside made me unrecognizable to myself, and the prospect of living was scarier than dying. Even after recently enduring weeks in a Turkish treatment facility, beginning medication, cognitive behavioral therapy, eye movement desensitization and reprocessing (EMDR), and electroconvulsive therapy (ECT), I somehow found myself

19

back in the hospital. Only this time, it was worse. Suicidal thinking and planning led to my previous hospitalization while action preceded this one.

Had I not learned from my first hospitalization?

Psychiatrist and trauma expert Bessel van der Kolk explained why I couldn't.

> We now know that trauma compromises the brain area that communicates the physical, embodied feeling of being alive. These changes explain why traumatized individuals become hypervigilant to threat at the expense of spontaneously engaging in their day-to-day lives. They also help us understand why traumatized people so often keep repeating the same problems and have such trouble learning from experience. We now know that their behaviors are not the result of moral failings or signs of lack of willpower or bad character— they are caused by actual changes in the brain.[1]

History repeated itself because a shift in my brain happened. Trauma changes your ability to feel alive, which to the traumatized Christian, may be equated with feeling abandoned by God.

Everything in me felt rejected, and the pain felt as though it really would kill me. "That's the thing about depression: A human being can survive almost anything, as long as she sees the end in sight. But depression is so insidious, and it compounds daily, that it's impossible to ever see the end. The fog is like a cage without a key."[2]

I realized that while science was utilized to save my life, it wasn't bringing my soul out of the black pit of despair or producing in me the will to live. If depression was an illness, why did the medical treatment not eradicate it? I knew my mind felt stabilized, but something was missing. My fluid understanding of depression as a faith problem began to entertain the thought that it is only an illness.

My staunchly held beliefs not only flip-flopped between two extremes, but now were unraveling all together. I didn't know what to think anymore. In the hospital, I would stand in a single-file line of patients twice a day to receive medication. A peculiar emptiness filled the eyes of those around me. Medication was something I benefited from, but the remaining void curated a question in my searching mind: was empty, controlled sadness what the rest of my life would look like? I vividly remember entertaining the question: "If this is the best life will be, what's the point?" I cringe when I remember the defeat of that question. I wish I could go back and tell myself that it would get so much better. That I would eventually get the help I needed medically, and that God's Word and my relationship with Him would literally bring me back to life. That I would one day look at my husband and children with blinders removed and want nothing more than to enjoy life with them. But while hospitalized I couldn't imagine a future from the blinding pain.

In the hospital, I slept on a simple bed, used a community bathroom that looked like those seen in prisons on TV, and privacy was a luxury not given to us. There were no mirrors, shower curtains, shoelaces, toilet seats, belts, drawstrings, or anything else that someone could creatively use to hurt themselves or others with.

Boredom in that institution left me to wander the dark alleys of my mind, while the random blood-curdling screams of other patients jolted me back to reality. Each startling cry I heard echoed the silent screams in my own soul. I felt stripped of everything, and I found myself without a Bible yet again. I didn't want to read the Bible, but there was still a part of me that thought it might help.

I spent much of my time sitting among others, observing those around me. Some patients were being admitted with severe mental illnesses I knew nothing of. Seeing patients talking to themselves or appearing to change personalities was shocking. Other patients were coming off drugs, which was something my sheltered eyes had never seen. Occasionally, patients shared unsolicited details of their own suicide attempts with me, sending my mind back to the moments I hung suspended between life and death. It was emotionally demanding to be in the place that was supposed to help me.

One night, a roommate was placed in my room while I was fast asleep. That night I jolted awake, sleepy-eyed and confused, by a woman running from her bed across the room to the foot of my bed yelling, "I am not a child molester" in a frantic voice that was deep and masculine.

My heart raced as I squinted my eyes open, staring at a stranger looking at me. Suddenly, an entirely different personality appeared to take over her body as she apologized with a feminine air about her and returned to her bed mere feet from mine. I discreetly flipped over while judgmentally thinking how crazy she was.

But conviction painted the situation in a different light when I realized she and I were both hospitalized, in the same ward, and in the same room. In a moment of life-altering humiliation, I saw myself in a more accurate light. Perhaps my mental illness was different than hers, but there we were—both broken and in need of help.

Learning of my weakness was a common theme during this season of my life. God's training to recognize my weakness was a painful process, but also a prerequisite for embracing my humanity and living a life of reliance on His power through me. My roommate and I both being equally human, and both made in the image of God revealed to me that we were more alike than I wanted to admit.

After a few nights of sleeping in fear of her unpredictability, she was moved to isolation. Would that happen to me if I were to break down? I was terrified of myself and desperate not to feel lonelier than I already was. Didn't God see how alone I was?

It would take me years to sort through these questions with God, but now I see,

> The pain of loneliness is one way in which He wants to get our attention.
>
> We may be earnestly desiring to be obedient and holy. But we may be missing the fact that it is *here*, where we happen to be at this moment and not in another place or another time, that we may learn to love Him—here where it seems He is not at work, where His will seems obscure or frightening, where He is not doing what we expected Him to do, where He is most absent. Here and nowhere else is the appointed place. If faith does not go to work *here*, it will not go to work at all.[3]

How could I go from standing in churches, declaring what the Lord was doing among the nations, to a patient in a locked psychiatric ward on suicide watch? My life shifted from pulpits to prison, or so it felt, and from acclaimed to ashamed.

I didn't know why God would let all of this happen to me, but in God's faithfulness and mercy, He did not stop the painful experiences because His ways are not our ways. He was more concerned with refining my character to be like Jesus than He was with my earthly comfort. So the furnace of affliction may have painfully burned hot, but its flames were bright with hope. "God rescues the afflicted by their affliction; he instructs them by their torment" (Job 36:15 CSB).

It was perseverance through affliction that would, in essence, save me from affliction. My torment was training me to hear His voice in adversity. In the mental hospital, I received my manna, much like the Israelites in the wilderness. I was led to that very institution so that I could truly learn to love Him and obey Him.

God appointed that very place as the ground from which my faith would grow. And so, the trials continued, but so did His grace. I felt abandoned and forgotten, but as the Lord would soon reveal to me that I was exactly where I was supposed to be.

One evening, I was told by a nurse that two of my friends were coming to visit. While waiting, there was nothing to distract me from the shame that made me want to hide, which is one of shame's traits. "Shame leads us to cloak ourselves with invisibility to prevent further intensification of the emotion."[4] I sat fidgeting, wondering how I would handle their assumed disappointment.

> When we experience shame, we tend to turn away from others because the prospect of being seen or known by another carries the anticipation of shame being intensified or reactivated. However, the very act of turning away, while temporarily protecting and relieving us from our feeling (and the gaze of the "other"), ironically simultaneously reinforces the very shame we are attempting to avoid. Notably, we do not necessarily realize this to be happening—we're just trying to survive the moment. But indeed, this dance between hiding and feeling shame itself becomes a tightening of the noose. We feel shame, and then feel shame for feeling shame. It begets itself.[5]

Waves of shame crashed into me as I saw the doors inched open. Then I saw Jamy enter, followed by my friend Necoe.

When I saw them walk through the door, varied feelings clashed within my heart, creating an emotional tornado. I couldn't decide if I should hug them or turn around and hide.

As Jamy sat next to me, I cringed inside knowing she was looking at me. Shame weighted my head making it a struggle to look up into her eyes. With no makeup on to hide my weariness, no hairbrush to tame my wild hair, and the way my pajamas awkwardly hugged my body due to weight gain from lifesaving medication, I was mortified. I couldn't manufacture joy or muster up any praises of God to try to impress her with. She was seeing me unedited and raw.

And it terrified me.

I appeared to be engaged in our small talk, but my mind entertained worries that she might walk away from me if she found out the secrets that I held tightly to for so many years. I did not take her decade-long investment in my life lightly. I was convinced, however, that she would see me as a waste of time, ultimately abandoning me because we weren't even biological family.

My insecurity with her flowed from my insecurity with God. I was absorbing lies from the enemy like a sponge, completely neglecting the fact that she came. She didn't have to, but she did.

This shame that was threatening my relationship was an ancient scheme straight from the depths of hell. The serpent's deception of Adam and Eve in the Garden of Eden enveloped them in shame as they hid from God. "The man and his wife heard the sound of the Lord God as he was walking in the garden in the cool of the day, and they hid from the Lord God among the trees of the garden. But the Lord God called to the man, 'Where are you?' He answered, 'I heard you in the garden, and I was afraid because I was naked; so I hid'" (Genesis 3:8–10). Like Adam and Eve, I felt naked sitting there.

> One of shame's most prominent features, and one that provides the emotional fuel of terror at the prospect of living vulnerably, is the threat of isolation, of abandonment. Our brains are wired with a deep suspicion of anything that might leave us alone in the ultimate sense. Thus, we are reluctant to expose ourselves, fearful that in doing so we may, once connected, be left.[6]

My terror melted into wonder as my insecurity was being challenged by her presence in that hospital. Jamy loved Jesus and lived unbound in the truth that God will never leave His children. Her faithfulness to me was an overflow of the Spirit within her. My relationship with her would be a vehicle God would use to help me believe the promise that He has not left us as orphans.

I met Jamy when I was a young mom in my twenties in Oklahoma where I lived as a newlywed. She was the pastor's wife and I eventually found the courage to attend her weekday Bible study. I felt out of place compared to the other ladies who knew the Bible well, but I was continually drawn back by Jamy's contagious love of Scripture. Without a mother's guidance, I blindly walked through those early years of marriage and motherhood. The more I learned about Jamy, the more I realized how much I could learn from her steady faith and living hope.

Eventually, I started lingering after her Bible study, asking her advice about various things. It happened so organically that I didn't even realize the Lord was knitting my heart to hers. As the years passed, she went from teacher to mentor to a spiritual mother who was raising me up in the faith.

Because I was dear to her, she shared not only the gospel of God with me, but her very life (1 Thessalonians 2:8). What bonded us together was our common commitment to Jesus. We shared the same reference point, and from our love of God, grew an affection for each other. It was all for Him, through Him, because of Him, and sustained by Him. "Focusing on God's glory gives beauty and depth to the spiritual mother-daughter relationship. The mutual desire to live for God's glory makes the relationship work."[7] Because her desire was to help cultivate in me a fruit bearing life that honored the Lord, my desire became that too. But that also made me so afraid to see her in my current condition.

What led to our embrace in that hospital was years in the making. She was there for me when my dad died. She was there for me when I nearly lost my life in childbirth. She rejoiced with me, and she wept with me. She listened to me, loved me, and never acted shocked by anything that came out of my mouth, creating a safe haven for me to be myself. She knew I struggled deeply, yet she did not give up on me.

"As the threads of lives are knit together, they become so interwoven that an environment of security is created."[8] Her steadfast love for me created the safety I needed to finally invite her into the unedited parts of my life. Being loved by her taught me that "the security of the relationship becomes a safer place than the aloneness of the cave."[9]

While sitting next to Jamy, I remember awkwardly mumbling something about my attempt to take my life. Suicide entered our conversation before I was ready. I felt vulnerable, exposed, and as I timidly looked up at Jamy's eyes, she looked right back at me. She was there because she loved me, not because of my behavior. That love is not only a reflection of the love of Christ, but it is safe.

"Traumatized human beings recover in the context of relationships: with families, loved ones, AA meetings, veterans' organizations, religious communities, or professional therapists. The role of those relationships is to provide physical and emotional safety."[10]

The pain of facing my actions, within the safety of family in Christ, was a necessary step in processing all that happened, specifically my attempt at suicide. That safety also gave me the courage to eventually turn around and face my future with hope and bravery. I saw that my friends didn't leave.

With no familial ties between us, there was really no obligation for her to stay. Because she chose to regardless of biology, a new hope challenged despair for center stage in my mind. I started to believe in that moment that maybe God hadn't left me either.

My friend, Necoe, who sat on the other side of the table as Jamy and me, bravely spoke Scripture to me. She reminded me that like the psalmist in Psalm 23:4, I was walking through the valley of the shadow of death. I hadn't considered Scripture much since being admitted to the hospital. I was merely trying to survive, not allowing much room for anything else to capture my attention. As Scripture pierced my heart, a flicker of truth turned into a small flame of hope. God softened my heart to hear the truth my friend reminded me of, and instead of salt on my emotional wounds, it was a healing balm.

Oftentimes people don't know what to do with a depressed loved one. Loving them can feel fruitless, but God is always at work doing more than we could ever ask or imagine. Jamy and Necoe knew the Bible well and could have preached at me, addressing the glaring issues in my life with Scripture.

But there is a time and a place for everything. By the leading of the Holy Spirit, they knew what I needed in that moment was a taste of hope and tangible love, even if I was incapable of reciprocating.

When a depressed believer feels the camaraderie of other believers, strength emerges, and healing begins. Their Christlike love only validated what science tells us: "Study after study shows that having a good support network constitutes the single most powerful protection against becoming traumatized. . . . When we are terrified, nothing calms us down like the reassuring voice or the firm embrace of someone we trust. Frightened adults respond to the same comforts as a terrified child."[11]

Just before visitors left, I remember insecurely asking Jamy to pray for me. She held my hands, grounding me with her comfort. As we sat among other patients in an extremely awkward setting, she prayed over me out loud. She didn't say sure and then leave me wondering if she ever actually did. She tucked me in as she raised her shield of faith over us both and confidently went to the throne of grace in my great time of need. Little did I know that her prayer was ushering in the very presence of God. He was restoring my soul, and it began with the obedience of other believers surrounding me with resolve that they wouldn't let me go down without a fight.

After they left, I joined the other patients in a common room. I sat in front of the TV when a patient, who was visibly detoxing from drugs, stood and walked right past me. As her legs brushed mine, she said out loud with great confidence "I will fear no evil, for you are with me" and kept walking. To my surprise, she quoted the next part of Psalm 23:4 that Necoe encouraged me with only moments before. I looked around to see if anyone else heard her declaration, but no one else was around.

I went back over the words in my mind: "Even though I walk through the valley of the shadow of death, I will fear no evil, for you are with me" (Psalm 23:4 ESV).

The fog of despair that consumed my mind suddenly began to dissipate and I knew the Lord was speaking. He was reminding me that I might be in a dark valley, but that I could fear no evil, for He was with me. My inability to have a Bible in the hospital did not stop God from using Scripture to transform my thinking. Miraculously hearing Scripture for the second time in the hospital was filling my weary soul with new life.

The next morning, and only a few days into my stay in this hospital, my turn had come to finally see the doctor for the first time. Without any idea that I was a Christian or about my encounter with Psalm 23 the day prior, the first thing he said was, "Julie, have you ever read Psalm 23?"

I could not believe it! God was reminding me yet again of the beautiful truth found in this beloved Psalm. There is no place so dark, so isolated, so removed from society that God cannot reach His children still. He was proving to be my Shepherd and he was providing what was lacking in my life: Scripture. "The Lord is my shepherd, I lack nothing" (Psalm 23:1). He was restoring all of me that once wandered away. Even as other patients would scream or suffer in various ways, I could feel change happening deep within. "He makes me lie down in green pastures. He leads me beside still waters. He restores my soul" (Psalm 23:2–3 ESV).

I was receiving my first taste of the beauty that comes when we combine medical treatment with therapeutic help, all the while allowing the Holy Spirit to speak to us through the Word of God. I needed medical help to steady my brain and keep me alive, but those treatments only stabilized the physical side of me. We are incredibly complex creations, and there is a spiritual aspect of who I am that was being neglected in my treatments. Medicine was a good gift, but Jesus was my hope. As my perspective began to shift, I decided I needed to cooperate with doctors, but I was convinced that cooperating with God was now equally important.

Jesus takes care of us and tells us in Scripture that "I am the good shepherd. I know my own, and my own know me" (John 10:14 ESV). God knew me. God intentionally searched for me with care. He found me because there is nowhere I can hide from His loving gaze. He tenderly nourished me with His words, and as His sheep, I knew His voice and I followed Him.

Even with a broken brain, I communed with the God Who Sees. It wasn't that I finally prayed enough or was still enough, or even possessed enough faith, for I was weary and still quite focused on death. It was that in God's perfect timing He made Himself known and was making me lie down in the hospital, the green pasture, I was in. My Shepherd was miraculously restoring my soul in the chaos of my unchanged circumstances. My mind was still ill, but peace permeated my spirit.

> For thus says the Lord God: Behold, I, I myself will search for my sheep and will seek them out. As a shepherd seeks out his flock when he is among his sheep that have been scattered, so will I seek out my sheep, and I will rescue them from all places where they have been scattered on a day of clouds and thick darkness.
> (Ezekiel 34:11–12 ESV)

> I myself will be the shepherd of my sheep, and I myself will make them lie down, declares the Lord God. I will seek the lost, and I will bring back the strayed, and I will bind up the injured, and I will strengthen the weak.
> (Ezekiel 34:15–16 ESV)

My heart, which still throbbed with the pain of depression, was experiencing the simultaneous joy that comes from His Spirit that lives within me. The sorrow made the joy sweeter and the joy made the sorrow endurable. The marriage of joy and sorrow in my mind and heart suddenly made sense. I was weak with sorrow, but the joy of the Lord was my strength. He was providing the medical care I needed, and it was binding up my injuries. He was feeding my mind His Word and it was strengthening all that was weak in me. God was true to His Word by not abandoning me after all, and He has not abandoned you.

Mental illness captures the enemy's attention as if there is a target on our minds. When an illness creates in us a bent toward sadness, it doesn't take much for satan to twist all that we know with a few lies. Spiritual warfare and mental illness go hand-in-hand in luring one of God's sheep away from the fold. As my enemies, who nearly killed me, still lurked in the shadows, my Shepherd prepared a table before me. "You prepare a table before me in the presence of my enemies" (Psalm 23:5 ESV).

The journey ahead of me would be long and treacherous. My emotions would still fluctuate between hope and despair. That's part of the imperfect progress that accompanies learning to thrive as a child of the Most High who lives with the debilitating sickness found in many minds.

And that's OK. Here I am, several years later, and I am still learning this lesson. For some reason as I was writing this, I swiped over on my phone, and I was shown a "Feature" photo. It was a selfie from the evening I attempted to take my life and ended up in the hospital. I didn't even remember this photo existed and certainly would have deleted it. My five-year-old, with zero idea of the circumstances surrounding that photo, saw it and said, "Who is that girl?"

I was shocked by the sincerity of his question. "You don't know who that is?"

"She looks evil," he said.

"Really?"

After scrolling to another photo, I then scrolled back to my selfie and he said, "I don't like that picture. She's scary. She looks evil."

Tears welled and a chill ran through my body. I felt afraid and shaky. How could the son who adores me not recognize me? I was smiling in the photo, but my son's discernment saw past that. Spirit-led words came to mind that a fellow sister in Christ declared to me a few weeks ago when I met her for the first time. After briefly telling her my story, she boldly told me, "That's not on you anymore."

My son saw the girl enslaved to darkness in that photo and didn't recognize her. My new friend met the girl freed from those chains and did not hold back from speaking truth to a kindred stranger. The enemy's plan to induce flashbacks of darkness actually produced remembrance of sacred encouragement. Satan's plan was intercepted by the Spirit and led to God's glory. My prayer since beginning to talk transparently about mental health has been that God would save lives, that others would not feel so alone and begin to emerge from the shadows. "As for you, you meant evil against me, but God meant it for good, to bring it about that many people should be kept alive, as they are today" (Genesis 50:20 ESV).

"Do not fear, for I have redeemed you; I have called you by your name; you are mine. When you pass through the waters, I will be with you, and the rivers will not overwhelm you. When you walk through the fire, you will not be scorched, and the flame will not burn you" (Isaiah 43:1–2 CSB).

The Shepherd is with you in the valley of the shadow of death and He keeps you.

He is with you in the waters that He promises won't overwhelm you.

He is with you in the fire that He says won't burn you.

He is patient as we learn to follow Him anew once trauma or mental illness has changed the very makeup of our brains. All of heaven rejoices as He leaves the ninety-nine to search for you. Surely His goodness and mercy are following you, even on days you don't feel it, all the days of your life.

3

A Thorn in My Mind

While cleaning my eleven-year-old daughter's messy bedroom, I found a drawing that said, "My mom is in the hospital today and it is her second time. I'm so sad. Sad is the only thing I feel."

Her words gripped my heart with shame and I wondered if the depression I was living with was ruining her. Memories from the psychiatric hospital stay she was referencing flooded my mind, along with guilt and fear despite having been released and doing well. Although I found myself in an emotional storm, my hope in Christ would soon prove firm and secure. That's the thing about hope when it is in Jesus. "This hope [this confident assurance] we have as an anchor of the soul [it cannot slip and it cannot break down under whatever pressure bears upon it]" (Hebrews 6:19 AMP).

Her drawing led to a family discussion on my mental health, where we offered more details of what I was going through, but then also used the opportunity to shine light on the overall topic of mental health with this next generation we are raising under our roof. Embracing authenticity in my mothering felt foreign, but in order to change the legacy of undiscussed mental illness and suicide my dad unfortunately passed on to me, I was determined to have the conversations with my children. It's hard to be the one to change a family pattern, but God can do more than we ask or imagine. My daughter's response to our conversation, however, caught me off guard and shocked me to the core.

"I'm scared I'm going to end up like you," she timidly confessed. Tears threatened my composure and an unmistakable grief manifested from thin air. She wasn't being mean; she was being honest. I always dreamed of my children, particularly my daughters, wanting to be like me, but that dream became fragmented by her freshly admitted fear, which the enemy twisted as a thorn in my flesh.

In the weeks prior to my daughter's comments, questions remained in the back of my mind, but I knew that if I was to ever improve, getting back in God's Word would be the only way. I encountered my Shepherd in the week I spent in the isolated psychiatric hospital following a suicide attempt, where He fed me Scripture when I didn't have access to it, but now that I was back home, settling into my new normal, I knew it was time that I opened my Bible.

I didn't want to in the beginning, and honestly, depression produced a numbness in me where I felt nothing as my eyes skimmed the pages. Despite reading feeling laborious, God's grace gave me the ability and strength to revisit His Word day after day, until one day, I was absolutely captivated. Early in this journey, I read the familiar story of the thorn in Paul's flesh found in 2 Corinthians and experienced a shift deep within.

Paul begins chapter twelve by sharing of an incredible experience he had with God where he was caught up to the third heaven. He discloses in the text that although he doesn't know if it was in the body or out of the body, it was still such an extraordinary experience that he would have had every reason to boast. He then goes on to say:

For if I want to boast, I wouldn't be a fool, because I would be telling the truth. But I will spare you, so that no one can credit me with something beyond what he sees in me or hears from me, especially because of the extraordinary revelations. Therefore, so that I would not exalt myself, a thorn in the flesh was given to me, a messenger of Satan to torment me so that I would not exalt myself. Concerning this, I pleaded with the Lord three times that it would leave me. But he said to me, "My grace is sufficient for you, for my power is perfected in weakness." Therefore, I will most gladly boast all the more about my weaknesses, so that Christ's power may reside in me. (2 Corinthians 12:6–9 CSB).

"God ensured that Paul remained close to the frailty of his humanity with the constant, painful pressing of the thorn, (Gr. Skolops, 'sharp, pointed piece of wood, splinter,' representing an unspecified ailment; a hapax or word used only here in the New Testament."[1]

A thorn indicates a physical malady of some sort. A physically painful one at that. While scholars speculate what Paul's thorn must have been, the vagueness of it lends to a beautifully applicable idea that will resonate with a multitude of "thorns" people find themselves plagued with. Charles Spurgeon, a deeply loved pastor who suffered from depression describes Paul's plight as so:

A thorn is but a little thing, and indicates a painful, but not a killing trial—not a huge, crushing, overwhelming affliction, but a common matter; none the less painful, however, because common and insignificant. A thorn is a sharp thing which pricks, pierces, irritates, lacerates, festers, and causes endless pain and inconvenience. And yet it is almost a *secret* thing—not very apparent to anyone but the sufferer. Paul had a secret grief somewhere, I know not where, but near his heart, continually wherever he might be, irritating him, perpetually vexing him, and

> wounding him. . . . It was not a sword in the bones,
> or a galling arrow in the loins, but only a thorn, about
> which little could be said! Everyone knows, however,
> that a thorn is one of the most wretched intruders that
> can molest our foot or hand; those pains which are
> despised because they are seldom fatal, are frequently
> the source of the most intense anguish—toothache,
> headache, earache—what greater miseries are known to
> mortals? . . . And if it remains in the flesh it will generate
> inconceivable torture.[2]

While contemplating the thorn in Paul's flesh, I noticed immediately that he asked the Lord to remove it three times, and yet God chose that it remain. This led me to reflect on the glaring issue that remained in my life despite my begging God for relief: Major Depressive Disorder and Post-traumatic Stress Disorder.

Awe filled my heart, followed by the first steps toward acceptance of God's sovereignty over every detail in my life, including if and when mental illness would be written into my story, and whether or not it might remain.

I finally understood.

Mental illness was a thorn in my flesh, or rather, a thorn in my mind.

Illness in the mind is a continual reminder of the human limitations that are perpetually humbling, painfully constant, and dreadfully difficult to endure. It's oftentimes invisible and completely irritating. Mental illness most certainly can generate inconceivable torture but entertaining the idea that God intends it for a purpose intrigued me to shift my perspective.

When depression causes fatigue, I see how physically weak I am. When traumatic flashbacks arrest my peace, I am reminded of my emotional weakness. When the sorrow is so intense that trusting God feels nearly impossible, I understand my spiritual weakness.

Fleshly afflictions, including mental illness, from the enemy's perspective begin and end with torment. Each irritation of the thorn—each trigger of a memory or dark thought—that has been thrust deep in my flesh was a reminder of the trial I was going through. As Scripture met my questions head on, I began to wonder if equating mental illness to a thorn in the flesh could allow for fresh vision and understanding of how mental illness could actually be used for my good and God's glory. As my perspective changed, my pain was infused with purpose, resulting in joy coexisting with my ever-present sorrow. Accepting the thorn as allowed by God for His purposes freed me to cooperate with His plan rather than fight it. Resentment over my struggles was replaced with a reverence for God that brought me into willing submission to His plan.

I believe God could heal every sickness in your body, remove every difficulty, and abolish every affliction in your life, for "with God all things are possible" (Matthew 19:26 CSB). But what about those situations where you pray for deliverance, with steady faith attached to those cries for help, and yet still remain in the same circumstance day after day? If we resist the notion that God is sovereign over everything that happens, and if we demand healing from Him, then we can easily be faced with a crisis of faith, an attitude of angry entitlement, and bitterness that will poison everything and everyone around us when God's plans don't align with ours.

With a softened heart, ready to cooperate with the Lord, I continued looking deeply into Paul's thorn.

From the very beginning of 2 Corinthians 12, we learn of Paul's great revelations. Whether or not they were in the body or out of the body, Paul did not know, but he declared that God knew. Paul was given extraordinary revelations from God— revelations that God knew were sure to tempt Paul toward an attitude of pride. There it was again—pride. God graciously revealed pride to me in the facade hiding my inner pain.

I liked to believe that I would never really fall victim to suicide, but given that Christians unfortunately can, that was awfully prideful to think I was above that sin.

In the passage of Scripture where we learn about Paul's thorn, what really piqued my interest was that God chose pain as a way to prevent pride in his beloved follower. Pain was Paul's protection. Paul experienced something special with God, so special that God knew he would have been prone to conceit.

And is that any different for anyone else in ministry? No. I really don't think it is. Being called to serve the church is a sacred calling, but without the proper perspective that we are clay and God is the potter, the human heart, which is simply prone to pride, can crumble under your God-given ministry which can be devastating.

There is this phenomenon that can happen in the lives of those who minister to others. It truly doesn't matter if you are a senior pastor, a worship leader, a missionary, a Sunday school teacher, or even a mother at home discipling your children. Mental illness highlights human weakness, and when allowed by God in the life of someone serving others perhaps it's the gracious means He has chosen to protect them from craving the pedestal many unknowingly place them on. For pastors, along with the pulpit can come a dangerous craving for the praise of man, but when depression has cultivated humility in the pastor, praise of God becomes the goal. For missionaries come the comments about how amazing you are for having courage to live in sometimes dangerous places, but when depression humanizes the missionary, it's realized that they are normal people who are simply serving God in a different context. This is something we must grasp together: we are all human, all broken, and all in need of a savior. Every single one of us.

It's beautifully humble and brave to be secure enough in Christ to allow your weakness to be a platform that displays the glorious power of God, rather than a cause of insecurity that will stand in the way of you being fully used by God and Him receiving all the glory through your life.

Don't let pride poison your fruitfulness.

Dependency on God is an absolute prerequisite for true, Spirit-filled, Spirit-led ministry, and if depression is the school in which dependency can be learned, then depression has been a gift allowed by God, for your good, your ministry, your relationship with Jesus, your joy, and God's kingdom.

The world tells you that your weakness disqualifies you for ministry, but nothing has happened to you that has not first passed through the hand of the God who is good and does good (Psalm 119:68). If you are suffering, rest assured that nothing comes as a surprise to God. Instead of resisting suffering, what if we accepted it? What if we cooperated with it, determined not to waste it, but rather walk through it in a manner worthy of our calling?

You may not have any say-so in whether or not you live with mental illness, but you can choose whether you will glorify the Lord through it or give into satan's plan of silencing and sidelining you.

Sometimes dark seasons are allowed as a sacred time of preparation for all that the Lord has planned for our lives, "For we are his workmanship, created in Christ Jesus for good works, which God prepared ahead of time for us to do" (Ephesians 2:10 CSB).

Regarding a pastor who struggles with mental illness, the valley of the shadow of death is a hard place for a shepherd to be, but the treasures the true Shepherd teaches the shepherd in the darkness deepen his ministry and ability to care for the afflicted in a way that shines with supernatural power and compassion.

The same goes for a mother who is tasked with shepherding the hearts of her children. Depression can certainly complicate parenting, but is does not have to be the death of your joy or sense of purpose in parenthood. It can be a holy reminder of the Most High who has chosen you to love and raise your children, but not in your own strength. For we must remember God's response to Paul's pleading to remove the thorn: "My grace is sufficient for you, for my power is perfected in weakness" (2 Corinthians 12:9 CSB). God may allow a thorn in your life, but with that thorn will always come His endlessly sufficient grace upon grace.

While this may not apply to you, I do want to speak to parents for a moment. Fellow parents, you are not a burden. There were years I believe that I was. Truly believed. "How on earth could you believe that?" you might be asking. It sounds completely ridiculous. But to the struggling mind, it sounds like absolute truth. It's a lie that becomes a driving force behind irrational thoughts that drive a wedge between a parent and their calling to care for their children, and when the drift away happens, the lie only grows in power and believability. It's one of the enemy's tired schemes that deceives so easily.

No one can replace you as mom or dad in their hearts. Yes, life could go on without you, but your worth as their mother is more than you can even fathom. The fight to get healthy is worth it. The discipline of feeding your mind transforming Truth from Scripture will pay off. If you are believing that your life is of so little value that your loved ones would actually taste relief if you weren't here, hear me now: that is a lie from the pits of hell.

You matter.

Your calling as a parent matters.

And there is beauty for them to behold in your weakness.

Weakness isn't something we naturally want to celebrate, though. Society teaches us that it's the independent who are worthy of imitation and the self-sufficient who are successful. I used to feel this way. In fact, I loathed my weakness in the beginning stages of being treated for mental illness and navigating the intimidating task of mothering through the darkness.

I didn't think I needed help, I didn't ask for help, and hiding my weakness tricked even my own mind that I was successful at being a mother. Yes, my children were fed and safe and dare I say even happy, but I was missing the joy God desired for me to experience in this calling on my life.

After beginning medication, talking to therapists, and trying various medical treatments, I definitely saw some stabilization, but my frustration flourished amid my unanswered questions and resistance to accepting my weakness.

"Was God tempting Paul? I wondered?" No, God was not tempting Paul, for we know that "God cannot be tempted with evil, and he himself tempts no one," (James 1:13 ESV) but God is the one "knows the secrets of the heart," (Psalm 44:21 CSB), and He knows the inclinations and limitations of the human mind. But here is a little detail that really made me stop and ponder: the thorn didn't just happen. But rather, it was given.

Given.

That word challenged my anger at God for allowing trials, opening my eyes to see that God gave it on purpose. God could have just not given Paul the revelations, or he could give the revelations plus pain.

It appears that God chose the latter, for it was Paul who said, "Therefore, so that I would not exalt myself, a thorn in the flesh was given to me, a messenger of Satan to torment me so that I would not exalt myself" (2 Corinthians 12:7 CSB). Mere happenstance wasn't responsible for the thorn, for it was intentionally given. The way I see it, Paul was presented with two options: he could bow up against the thorn God chose to give him, or he could humbly accept the trial while believing God when He said: "For my thoughts are not your thoughts, and your ways are not my ways" (Isaiah 55:8 CSB).

And this is where I found solace in the mental illness God was not healing. It started with my acceptance, that is "the act of taking or receiving something offered" (dictionary.com), of that which God gave, rather than rebellion.

How could mental illness be good in my life? That perspective seemed illogical when pondered through the filter of faltering faith. But what if our human definition of "good" is not the divine definition of "good"? God allowing a messenger of satan to torment His beloved might seem especially cruel at first glance, but let's remember why the thorn was given. The thorn was given to defeat the sin that God knew would bubble up in Paul, so therefore God was using satan to defeat the very scheme of satan. It's brilliant if you think about it.

The mentally ill child of God lives with a keen awareness of their need for God, and when they see that God allowing satan's torment is a way to defeat satan, a feeling of gratefulness infiltrates grief. You become a beautiful arena where the war between satan and God is put on display for others to see. And God always wins; He's already won.

Through the transparency in which you live, people watching will be compelled to embrace their weakness as well, ultimately leading to God receiving glory on this earth. This is another example of purpose in your pain.

Look back at Paul's initial reaction to his thorn. He didn't find this "thorn" pleasant, as we know he pleaded with God to take it away three times.

> Three times I pleaded with the Lord to take it away from me. But he said to me, "My grace is sufficient for you, for my power is made perfect in weakness." Therefore I will boast all the more gladly about my weaknesses, so that Christ's power may rest on me. That is why, for Christ's sake, I delight in weaknesses, in insults, in hardships, in persecutions, in difficulties. For when I am weak, then I am strong. (2 Corinthians 12:8–10)

For a Christian, mental illness is certainly a humbling reminder of your humanity. Mental illness—this thorn in my flesh, or rather in my mind—has been allowed by God, as nothing can happen outside the knowledge and allowance of God. But what about the person enduring the torment of the thorn? What if we turned our inward gaze outward and remembered that it's not all about us?

The thorn isn't meant to bring shame upon us, but rather to shame the enemy of our souls and sabotage his plan. As a child of God, there will be a thorn in your flesh, for your understanding of your weakness in relation to God is just too important for God not to intervene by teaching us just how weak we are. So how are we supposed to respond to this thorn?

With gladness.

Paul wrote: "But he said to me, 'My grace is sufficient for you, for my power is perfected in weakness.' Therefore, I will most gladly boast all the more about my weaknesses, so that Christ's power may reside in me" (2 Corinthians 12:8–9).

Gladly (Greek: hedistos) has the idea of "Most sweetly, with great relish, when spoken of eating and drinking. In the NT, used figuratively in 2 Cor 12:9, 15, meaning most gladly."[3]

When Paul said, "I will most gladly boast all the more about my weaknesses" (2 Corinthians 12:9), he is saying he will boast with great relish, as if you were savoring your favorite dessert, and the Greek word *hedistos* is the opposite of the Greek word *Pikros*, which means "bitterly. Used of bitter weeping."[4]

When we look back at the account in the book of Matthew where Peter denies Jesus before His crucifixion, we find this word *pikros* (bitterly): "And Peter remembered the saying of Jesus, 'Before the rooster crows, you will deny me three times.' And he went out and wept bitterly [*pikros*]" (Matthew 26:75 ESV). Can you imagine the level of sadness that Peter felt just after denying the Son of God? That is an extremely bitter sadness.

Trials in life can harden your heart with bitterness or soften your heart with gladness, and the secret to choosing the latter is a perspective that embraces weakness for the glory of God and with the strength God's grace gives.

And so, in the moment where my daughter's confession brought sorrow, I finally felt the gladness Paul wrote about. My grief from hearing her words was infused with hope, shifting my perspective from the seen to the unseen. Hope and grief can coexist, and God's grace filled me with strength to continue parenting in that difficult moment.

God intervened by giving me spiritual eyes to see past my circumstances. There was beauty in the weakness my daughter saw in my life if it led to my daughter realizing the power of God in her mother and not her mother's perfection. My flesh wanted her to desire to be like me, but when God helped me realize through Scripture that her learning to be like Jesus was a more important goal. Therefore, boasting in my weakness with her became a platform for God's power to shine bright, calm her fears, and produce a sustaining gladness in my heart of hearts.

When hope mingles with our suffering, suddenly our pain is rich with purpose, and perseverance becomes possible when we stop fighting that which we don't understand, accepting our lot in life as part of God's greater plan. Can we still ask for healing and cry out to God for deliverance? Absolutely. The Bible is full of stories like this. But can we learn to embrace God's plan when it includes suffering? Yes, because the joy of the Lord really can be our strength as His grace sustains us in our sorrow. Our hearts glow with love for that which we esteem. When Jesus becomes our highest joy, we really can yearn for his glory and presence over our comfort and ease.

As I sat with my daughter, the wisdom of God helped me look forward to the future with confident expectation of God's faithfulness. I cast a vision of hope for my daughter by explaining to her that she won't end up like me, because God is redirecting the trajectory of our family line by changing me. I explained to her that every hospitalization has happened not in spite of her, but because He cares too much about His plan for her to allow suicide to continue to ravage this family. My dad's suicide increases the risk of me dying in the same manner, and the mental illness I live with certainly fuels that statistic. But statistics cannot stand up to God's power. You really can be the one to change the way a family has functioned for years.

As I spoke hope over my daughter, I felt the Father singing hope over me. But in one ear the enemy whispered that my illness was damaging her, yet I know her story will be used as a way to proclaim Christ.

Making the difficult decision to embrace my weakness in the pursuit of mental and spiritual health has been one of the most loving things I've done as her mother. My depression isn't ruining her, but rather refining her as it is me. When our children see their mom struggle, cry out to God, and the transformation that comes from faith in Christ, they see faith in action. They see the power of God's Word, and they see that it's OK to not be OK. Their own salvation story might even stem from the way Jesus shines through the brokenness in your own life.

God has a purpose in weaving mental illness through your story, for you are part of a bigger story that is ever-unfolding. It's for His glory that we suffer. It's for His glory that we endure. It's for His glory that we pass our living hope down to our children which is beautifully seen when we allow them to see His strength in our weakness.

Your fight for hope honors Jesus in a way that your children will remember when they too go through trials someday— trials that God chooses to use as a thorn in their flesh. If you hide every aspect of your suffering from them, how will they be ready to cling to hope in crisis and follow Him faithfully when everything seems dark?

It's OK to struggle. It's OK to share appropriate details with your children. Do not waste your suffering but rather use it as a way to point your children to Jesus. They are watching and craving authenticity rather than manufactured perfection. They adore you and will be more likely to cling to hope, even in the most horrific of times, if they see you do it first.

The trauma or mental illness you're thinking of as your thorn has not ruined your purpose. The way God has sustained you through it and the aftermath, including flashbacks and hypervigilance, might just be the very testimony from your life that will be used to save others for all of eternity. "Great comfort comes from understanding pain as a partnership with God. Suffering is a way to bring God glory. Trials are a way to show Him strong. Heartache is a way to demonstrate His sufficiency. Affliction is a way to experience His nearness. Acceptance is a way to bring Him pleasure. Isn't this life really about Him?"[5]

I've truly come to a place of acceptance with what is clearly God's will for my life at this time. When we receive both the good and the hard from our Father in heaven, our contentment will speak to others of God's all-sustaining grace. For even Job said in the midst of his suffering, "'Should we accept only good from God and not adversity?' Throughout all this Job did not sin in what he said" (Job 2:10 CSB). My daughter's story as my child has included pain, but my hope is that her life will shine with compassion for others from the hope-filled story God is giving her as my daughter.

As you consider what your thorn may be, my prayer over you is one of gladness, and that you'll adopt the words of David as your very own: "I saw the Lord always before me. Because he is at my right hand, I will not be shaken. Therefore my heart is glad and my tongue rejoices; my body also will rest in hope, because you will not abandon me to the realm of the dead, you will not let your holy one see decay. You have made known to me the paths of life; you will fill me with joy in your presence" (Acts 2:25–28).

Dying to yourself is essential in following Jesus. And if you've asked God for healing from mental illness, and have yet to receive it, we can only conclude that His will includes mental illness in your mortal body for the time being for purposes beyond our comprehension.

Dying to self may look like letting go of your idea of what your life should look like in exchange for what God has designed your life to be. When we grasp the sovereignty of God over every aspect of every single thing, and believe in His goodness and love for us, we can embrace our weakness as the beautiful design to display His strength and draw others to Him.

This is the beauty that comes from accepting suffering in your life as a Christian. Death might be at work in you, but life will be at work in those watching Jesus sustain you. And this is a reason for blazing hope and radiant joy in the midst of sorrowful suffering. The joy has an energizing power to then produce endurance in the race you've been called to run with purpose. Depression, anxiety, bipolar disorder, along with any other mental illness you might be struggling with, may be producing suicidal thoughts—death in you—but when you learn to say no, which is often where therapy comes into play, and choose to cling to Christ as you wait for the tumultuous emotions to subside, then life will be at work in others who see the Lord sustaining you. Like Paul said to the Corinthians, "So then, death is at work in us, but life in you" (2 Corinthians 4:12 CSB).

When mental illness is a thorn in the flesh of a Saint, the daily struggles are often a hidden battle with death that others can't see. But remember this: "Though our bodies are dying, our spirits are being renewed every day. For our present troubles are small and won't last very long. Yet they produce for us a glory that vastly outweighs them and will last forever! So we don't look at the troubles we can see now; rather we fix our gaze on things that cannot be seen. For the things we see now will soon be gone, but the things we cannot see will last forever" (2 Corinthians 4:16–18 NLT).

4

Sober-Minded

I remember several years before we returned to the US a moment when cars came at us from every side as we dashed across the busy road near our Central Asian home. Their physical threat, however, was small in comparison to the joy-threatening lies of the enemy that accompanied my young son's sudden question.

"Mom, we are mad at your dad, aren't we?" he asked me at what seemed like the most inopportune time.

But really, is there ever a good time to address such difficult and grief laden questions? My son realized that his grandpa died by suicide later in his life since he was too young to understand the method when the death actually took place. His inquiry was innocent and insecure. I heard his "we" and realized my feelings toward my father, whose suicide left me parentless, were about to be adopted by my ten-year-old son.

"Lord, help me," I prayed silently as my dread of this conversation created a lump in my throat. That prayer was all I could produce, but it was enough for God to intervene and help me see the situation through a filter of faith rather than the emotional fog that was attempting to cloud my vision.

Although time marched forward as we walked on the busy road, it seemed to stand still as his question caught me off guard. Suppressed memories flashed through my mind and my heart tasted the bitterness of old questions and labels I fight daily with my shield of faith, for Scripture tells us "In all circumstances take up the shield of faith, with which you can extinguish all the flaming darts of the evil one" (Ephesians 6:16 ESV).

Abandoned. Orphaned. Alone. Unwanted. Unlovable. Angry.

Bitter.

Irrational thoughts and flashbacks beat my mind with hurricane-like force. These identities I'm tempted to wear, were suddenly brought to light by the Spirit as the chains of bondage that they really are. Chains my son was about to pick up. Chains that are strong but snap like thread when exposed to the precious promises God has given us—promises He has given me the discipline to cling to; promises that must be learned in order to hide behind; promises that promote a sober mind; promises that do not fail in the heat of the Refiner's Fire.

I was able to transition our conversation into one that created mercy in my son rather than hatred. When we learn to mourn the losses of those who die by suicide and take the time to understand the way illness can lead to such an irrational action, then we are able to look at the person with compassion rather than bitterness. Even a Christian who loves Jesus can make such a devastating decision in the heat of the moment if they let their guard down for even one second.

Does my heart still ache? Yes. Do I still get upset and feel forsaken? Of course. But over time, reading God's Word while also receiving help from therapy has taught me how to step outside of the emotion and see my dad's devastating decision with grace. And while this is not always easy, with God, it is possible.

At one time I was so afraid of my dark emotions and the enemy's power, but confidence in God as my Protector has grown through each small moment of deliverance where I have turned to Him in desperation rather than away from Him in depression. I can honestly look to God today and say, "The Lord is my light and my salvation; whom shall I fear? The Lord is the stronghold of my life; of whom shall I be afraid?" (Psalm 27:1 ESV).

And while perhaps this situation was handled as it should have been with my son on that busy Central Asian road, and my sober mind could function apart from my emotion or miraculously in spite of my illness, it wasn't always so.

Whether it's excessive worry because of anxiety, racing thoughts because of bipolar disorder, or suicidal thoughts that can often accompany depression, many illnesses certainly include something related to thoughts.

For example, according to the DSM-5, the manual used by psychiatrists in treating patients, when looking at the diagnostic features of Major Depressive Disorder, "Thoughts of death, suicidal ideation, or suicide attempts are common. They may range from a passive wish not to awaken in the morning or a belief that others would be better off if the individual were dead, to transient but recurrent thoughts of committing suicide, to a specific suicide plan."[1]

While living with a mental disorder certainly makes it difficult to objectively look at our own thoughts and understand their irrationality, it's not impossible for the mind that is being transformed and renewed by Scripture. It might not come easily at first, but we must remember to not neglect the Word of God. We find mental sobriety when we follow Scripture that tells us, "but be transformed by the renewing of your mind, so that you may discern what is the good, pleasing, and perfect will of God" (Romans 12:2 CSB).

What we allow our minds to focus on matters, but sometimes we might not fully understand the danger of the thoughts swirling inside our minds, hidden from the outside world, but very real to you and completely exposed to God, until it's too late. Those fleeting thoughts that don't seem to pose a threat like "Maybe I just won't wake up in the morning," or "Maybe I'll happen to get in a car wreck and die," are worthy of notice. Those hidden desires like "I wish I could just get sick and die," are screaming for attention. Thoughts of that nature reveal weariness and sadness in your life, but maybe you don't feel the urgency to address them since you believe that there are no actual plans attached to those thoughts.

However, those desires and thoughts left unattended can drag you into evil and lure you away into darkness. The thoughts and desires that you are struggling with at this very moment may seem harmless, but evil thoughts give birth to evil actions, and when sin is allowed to grow, it gives birth to death. "And remember, when you are being tempted, do not say, 'God is tempting me.' God is never tempted to do wrong, and he never tempts anyone else. Temptation comes from our own desires, which entice us and drag us away. These desires give birth to sinful actions. And when sin is allowed to grow, it gives birth to death" (James 1:13–15 NLT).

Desire isn't necessarily a bad thing, but rather "Describes a strong, deep-seated desire or longing for anything—good or bad. However, when that desire grows out of control and becomes a governing habit, the bent toward sinning takes charge. Clearly the fault for inappropriate 'desires' rests entirely with the individual. God cannot be blamed. Then human desire becomes so overwhelming that you overlook or ignore the trap until there is no turning back."[2]

Your thoughts have the power to draw you away, even you, dear Christian who loves Jesus and wants to live a life worthy of all that you've been called to. When James 1:14 mentions "drag away" or "draw away," it's the Greek word *exelkomenos*. "It's a hunting term used to describe a trap designed to lure and catch an unsuspecting animal."³ The word "lure" in Greek is "a term suggesting luring prey from safety to capture and even death."⁴

This passage in the book of James reminds us that God tests his people (for example, Abraham [Genesis 22]; Israel [Exodus 16:4]; Hezekiah [2 Chronicles 32:31]) so that their character is strengthened, but he never tempts (for example, lures people into sin). Since God cannot be tempted with evil, and He is unreservedly good, He would never entice human beings to sin or seek to harm their faith. Tempted (Gk. *peirazo*) is a verb form of the noun translated "trial" (Gk. *peirasmos*) in James 1:12, but the context shows that different senses of the word are intended. God brings trials in order to strengthen the Christian's faith.

He never tempts, however, because he never desires his people to sin. Christians should never blame God when they do wrong (ESV Study Bible on James 1:13), and so when we feel the intrusive thoughts tempt us toward escape, we can never blame God for them. Each difficult aspect of living with a mental illness is a trial, but it's not a trial without purpose for your good. Therefore, "Consider it a great joy, my brothers and sisters, whenever you experience various trials, because you know that the testing of your faith produces endurance. And let endurance have its full effect, so that you may be mature and complete, lacking nothing" (James 1:2–4 CSB).

But as you endure, I know the thoughts might continue. The thoughts inside your mind that come out of nowhere and have great emotion attached to them. These thoughts are intrusive, dangerous, and have the power to lure and entice you when your emotions become dictators instead of mere indicators.

James uses a fishing metaphor to illustrate the act of drawing prey away from their safe shelter in order to capture and trap them with a hook that proves deadly. Here, James talks about how it is the person's own evil desire that ensnares them.

Following the fishing metaphor, "The picture changes to a birth/rebirth metaphor, as full-grown desire bears its own child, sin, which itself grows into maturity and bears the grandchild, death. This dramatic depiction shows the terrible result when one gives in to temptation."[5]

How sad is that metaphor? Maybe you've lost a child, and if so, this will particularly hit very close to home in the most heartbreaking of ways. When you're pregnant, you long to meet your baby. The pregnancy is full of hopeful expectation, and you see the end as nothing but joy.

After all the labor pains, instead of a joyful life being placed in your arms, sorrowful death comes over the long-awaited child you now stare at with a shattered heart. Sin is the same. It offers pleasure, but ends in loss. The intrusive thoughts that tempt you to escape your pain entice you by offering relief from pain, but in reality, nothing but destruction and immense sorrow is present after the horrid act is committed.

As a Christian, perhaps you personally would not be in pain anymore, but everyone left would be in absolute devastation, and your fruitfulness as a Christian on earth would be stolen from you. The belief that suicide is the courageous choice that will end pain is irrational because suicide multiplies pain and destroys lives. I can say with confidence that no one—and I repeat no one—will taste relief at your passing. Questions will haunt the survivors most likely every day of their time left on earth. Many will feel guilty, going over every last interaction with you to see if there was some way they could have stopped you.

Again, your mind matters, as Jesus said, "Love the Lord your God with all your heart and with all your soul and with all your mind. This is the first and greatest commandment" (Matthew 22:37–38). Because satan will stop at nothing to hinder you from living out this command, and he knows your flesh is bent toward sin, he celebrates the war zone hidden away in your mind. Going directly for the part of us that controls so much of our behavior and beliefs is genius on his part and understandably one of his schemes. He knows your soul is secure and is fully aware that Jesus was speaking of those who belong to Him when we said, "My Father, who has given them to me, is greater than all, no one can snatch them out of my Father's hand. I and the Father are one" (John 10:29–30). So what does the enemy do? He goes after those sinful desires that come from your sinful nature, and he is ruthless in destroying your beautiful witness to this world. He loves your irrational thoughts and will use them against you.

Irrational thoughts often accompany mental illness, so much so that the enemy can cleverly capture believers in a web of lies and wrong thinking without much effort on his part. Fallacious thoughts seem factual inside a mind that exists in a fallen world.

What's scary is that desperate despair can glamorize the giving up on life, creating the illusion of courage in the one who can carry it out. Suicide seems like a sensible choice when the mind is not sound, but that delusive glamour never delivers relief to those who you believe you are a burden on. That deceitfulness of sin leaves destruction in its path. This is not God's will for your life and legacy. Suicide will never be God's desire for you.

We cannot grow lax in fighting the good fight for our minds. Our minds matter too much and play too big a part in our ability to shine for Christ for us to allow ourselves to become "drunk" so to speak when it comes to the spiritual truth that God has graciously given us in His Word. Believers, even mentally ill ones, are meant to live in the light of Christ, not the pitch-black darkness ruled by satan.

We find this truth in 1 Thessalonians 5:5–8 (ESV),

> For you are all children of light, children of the day. We are not of the night or of the darkness. So then let us not

sleep, as others do, but let us keep awake and be sober.
For those who sleep, sleep at night, and those who get
drunk, are drunk at night. But since we belong to the
day, let us be sober, having put on the breastplate of
faith and love, and for a helmet the hope of salvation.

"The idea of sober in this context includes spiritual
stability, stability we need in Christ, in the Spirit, to withstand
the onslaught of the darkness. As the return of Christ draws
nigh, and the temptations of darkness intensify, it is absolutely
crucial for believers to have a cool collected, mind of Christ
attitude toward temptation."[6]

You can never forget who you are in Christ as a born-again
believer. Regardless of whether or not you live with a mental
illness, you are a child of light and child of the day. In Romans
13:11–12 (CSB), Paul tells believers to "wake up from sleep,
because now our salvation is nearer than when we first believed.
The night is nearly over, and the day is near; so let us discard
the deeds of darkness and put on the armor of light."

One of the enemy's great strategies is to nurture the
sleepiness of saints. You were not called to sleep through life,
but rather to walk fully awake and sober minded. Trauma from
your past may throw you headlong into a trance leaving you
feeling as though you are being moved around in life with a
sleepy lethargy that can be equated to sleep walking, but God
is greater than the tyranny of trauma.

Depression can feel so demanding that sleeping your day
away literally, or spiritually, is easier than fighting the weary
emotions that accompany such a difficult illness. But you,
beloved saint, were meant for so much more. "The night is
nearly over; the day is almost here. So let us put aside the deeds
of darkness and put on the armor of light" (Romans 13:12).
You are "to take off your former way of life, the old self that
is corrupted by deceitful desires, to be renewed in the spirit
of your minds, and to put on the new self, the one created

according to God's likeness in righteousness and purity of the truth" (Ephesians 4:22–24 CSB).

There is action required, and mental illness certainly has no bearing over whether or not you must obey. You must "put on the Lord Jesus Christ, and make no provision for the flesh to gratify its desires" (Romans 13:14 CSB). You must put on Christ so that you won't fall into the trap of thinking ahead and planning sin. To be frank, fumbling around in the darkness of depression, not actively renewing the mind with Scripture, and not living in complete dependence on Him, yet still claiming to be a Christian might not be much more than using religion to cover your old self.

In Christ, you are a new creation who has been not only transformed but transferred from the kingdom of darkness to the kingdom of light. Your relationship with Him gives life and victory. You are to watch and pray and fling off any sin that easily entangles you.

There must be a hatred and renouncement of sin and a putting on of the armor of Light as the way to thrive as a child of God who lives with mental illness. You cannot make any provision, or plan ahead, for your flesh to give into its sinful desires.

Researching, learning, and planning ways to indulge the sinfulness that can stem from mental illness, such as making a plan for suicide or self-harm, is not living out Romans 13:14, so therefore put on the Lord Jesus Christ, and allow His presence to envelop you as you abide in Him. You, child of Light and child of the day, are meant to live in wholeness even if your mind is broken by illness.

You are meant for joy despite your sorrow, and triumph even after trauma. Fling off the deeds of darkness once and for all, or rather rip them off with all your might and run with radiance rather than limp in shame. Because your Shepherd will never forsake you, you can forsake the sinful darkness that you are tempted to indulge in. Putting on Christ is the same as embracing His values and putting on His characteristics. Putting on Christ is not a burden, but rather your protection.

Maybe like I once did, you're wondering how a Christian can live with a sober mind as Scripture clearly teaches when they battle a mental illness? How do they live in the Light when they are drawn to the dark. A sober mind with a mental illness almost seems like an impossible thing, but take heart, it's not. Yes, mental illness is a real illness that can impede the metal facilities, but nothing, and I repeat, nothing is too hard for our God.

The Bible says, "Be sober-minded, be alert. Your adversary the devil is prowling around like a roaring lion, looking for anyone he can devour" (1 Peter 5:8 CSB).

"Therefore, with your minds ready for action, be sober-minded and set your hope completely on the grace to be brought to you at the revelation of Jesus Christ" (1 Peter 1:13 CSB).

"The end of all things is near; therefore, be alert and sober-minded for prayer" (1 Peter 4:7 CSB).

We are told over and over in Scripture to be sober-minded, but an illness that brings with it irrational thoughts can defeat the Christian who is not vigilant and awake.

But what does it really mean to be sober (Greek: *nepho*)?

> The NT (New Testament) uses nepho only in the figurative sense meaning to be free from every form of mental and spiritual "intoxication." The idea is to be calm and collected in spirit, circumspect, self-controlled, well-balanced, clear headed. Be self-possessed ("Spirit" possessed) under all circumstances. Nepho speaks of exercising self-restraint (enabled by the Spirit) and being free from excess, from evil passion, from rashness, etc. Without sobriety true vigilance is impossible.
>
> And so Paul is calling believers to continually (present tense) live soberly and in this state we are more alert and watchful and less likely of being enticed by

the deeds of darkness. Night people can only do night deeds and cannot do the deeds of the day. However sons of light and sons of day can do the deeds of the night, tracking back to their old patterns of conduct. To be sure, as sons of day we have the power to commit sins, but we can still commit acts of darkness unless we remain sober. What is even more tragic is that when believers commit sins, they do so in the light of God's revealed truth, regarding our dethroned sinful nature. Paul calls for our behavior to be consistent with our new nature.[7]

Sober (*nepho*) can be seen as the antithesis of irrational thinking. To be sober is to be stable, unwavering, and steadfast. To be sober-minded is to think clearly and be fully aware and awake of what is going on in your mind, so you can correctly evaluate the thoughts that appear out of nowhere and make the right choice to flee from those thought's commands rather than indulge them.

But sometimes it feels impossible to escape the suicidal thoughts, and perhaps that's because you have an enemy who strategically uses your natural inclination toward rebellious thoughts as a way to lure you into his stronghold, and when I say stronghold, I'm not referring to an occasional, random thought or sin. I'm referring to a thought pattern or sin that has become habitual and so second nature that you believe it's impossible to even separate yourself from it.

When a certain thought becomes engrained in your mind, it becomes easy to believe it's your identity and at the core of who you really are.

A stronghold is a thought pattern that forms a fortress around the mind, holding it prisoner to faulty thinking. It is formed brick-by-brick by repetitive faulty thinking or all at once by a onetime traumatic event such as a rape, molestation, or abuse.

In the Old Testament, a stronghold was a fortified dwelling used for protection from an enemy. David hid in wilderness strongholds when he was hiding from King Saul, who was trying to kill him (1 Samuel 22:4; 23:14). These were usually caves high on a mountainside or some other structure that was hard to attack. In the Old Testament, God is called our stronghold: "The Lord is a refuge for the oppressed, a stronghold in times of trouble" (Psalm 9:9).

"The New Testament writers took this same imagery of a fortress to describe the spiritual tower of bondage, not protection, that we put ourselves in by developing thought patterns and ideas that hold us captive. . . . It is anything that sets itself up against the knowledge of God. A stronghold does not protect us, it protects the enemy who is manipulating our thoughts and suggesting our actions."[8]

I love how Pastor Steve Berger describes a stronghold as "A satanic lie, a generational mindset or a human wounding that you have listened to long enough, believed strongly enough, and owned deeply enough that it becomes part of your identity. It has fortified itself in you and dictates your thoughts, beliefs, actions and reactions. It is an unholy filter through which all thoughts pass."[9]

Satan knows how important the mind is and understands that whatever controls the mind becomes the master of one's thoughts and actions. The mind is a very strategic place for the enemy to capture, especially since our desires naturally draw us away from Christ. But you, Child of God, are not meant to be a prisoner in the enemy's stronghold or a victim of your own desires, for you belong to Jesus and are called to live according to the Spirit.

"Those who are dominated by the sinful nature think about sinful things, but those who are controlled by the Holy Spirit think about thinks that please the Spirit. So letting your sinful nature control your mind leads to death. But letting the Spirit control your mind leads to life and peace" (Romans 8:5–6 NLT).

To set your mind on the flesh means you habitually focus on and desire things that are characteristic of the sinful human nature that Jesus has rescued you from. Continually thinking about things that are sinful is an indication that you are not walking in the identity that is yours through Christ Jesus, but rather thinking the same way as the unbelieving world thinks. "So if you have been raised with Christ, seek the things above, where Christ is, seated at the right hand of God. Set your minds on things above, not on earthly things. For you died, and your life is hidden with Christ in God" (Colossians 3:1–3 CSB).

Setting your mind on things above is an action that requires obedience. Savoring the intrusive thoughts that plague your mind is an act of rebellion. Yes, I said it, rebellion. Through the blood of Christ, you are a new creation, full of the same power that resurrected Jesus from the grave. You are not helpless in your habitual, suicidal thoughts. I know it feels that way, but feelings are known for telling lies. Our affections matter, and when they are tainted by sin and sickness, they can tenderly attach themselves to thoughts that a child of God has no place entertaining.

> Seeking the things above is not mysticism or mere "positive thinking," "visualization," or "mind over matter." It is however true that a as a man thinks in his heart, so he is. And so as he surrenders to the Spirit and partakes of grace to enable him to seek the heavenly things, his mind is renewed and is less likely to choose the base and profane things of this world. A powerful way to aid our seeking the things above is to memorize the Word of God which speaks about the things above. Then we will be able to recall those heavenly truths to mind no matter where we find ourselves during the day.[10]

Let's look at the book of Philippians together, which is a letter penned by the apostle Paul to the church at Philippi, from prison. "The chief theme of Philippians is encouragement. Paul wants to encourage the Philippians to live out their lives as citizens of a heavenly colony, as evidenced by a growing commitment to service to God, and to one another. The way of life that Paul encourages was manifested uniquely in Jesus Christ."[11]

Near the end of the letter, Paul encourages the Philippians by instructing them what to set their minds on: "And now, dear brothers and sisters, one final thing. Fix your thoughts on what is true, and honorable, and right, and pure, and lovely, and admirable. Think about things that are excellent and worthy of praise. Keep putting into practice all you learned and received from me—everything you heard from me and saw me doing. Then the God of peace will be with you" (Philippians 4:8–9 NLT).

Anxiety is a condition of the mind, and how many of us know what anxiety feels like? It can feel like an overwhelming burden that both scares and exhausts those who live with it. You are not helpless though, since the Helper lives in you. "For God is working in you, giving you the desire and the power to do what pleases him" (Philippians 2:13 NLT).

> The human mind will always set itself on something and Paul wished to be quite sure that the Philippians would set their minds on the right things. This is something of the utmost importance, because it is a law of life that, if a man thinks of something often enough, he will come to the stage when he cannot stop thinking about it. His thoughts will be quite literally in a groove out of which he cannot jerk them. It is, therefore, of the first importance that a man should set his thoughts upon the fine things and here Paul makes a list of them.[12]

So, let's break it down.

To think on whatever is true is important because the spiritual battle is essentially a truth struggle, with our mind and heart being the place the battle rages daily. In order to remain spiritually stable, we must stand on the truth and we must do that every day. So what is the truth?

It is the Word of God, for Jesus asked the Father to "Sanctify them by the truth; your word is truth" (John 17:17) when praying about believers before His death. The truth is the force that will dismantle the lies that the enemy tells you. From the beginning of time, lies and deception have been a tactic of satan as seen when he injected doubt about God's Word to Adam and Eve followed by an outright lie. To know the truth will keep your mind sober when lies are being whispered in your ear.

To think on whatever is honorable is to think about that which will inspire awe and reverence. When a believer meditates on that which is temporal or earthly instead of focusing on all that is heavenly and worthy of praise, their mind will have a greater eternal perspective. All that is in God's Word is certainly honorable and should be thought on.

To think on what is right is to think on all that is perfectly in harmony with the standards God reveals to us in Scripture. "In the NT those that are called righteous (*dikaioi*) are those who have conditioned their lives by the standard which is not theirs, but God's. They are the people related to God and who, as a result of this relationship, walk with God."[13]

To think on what is pure is to think on that which is innocent, pure, blameless, and free from impurities and defilement. Jesus Himself is pure, so we must take every thought and ask ourselves, "Does this thought make me more like Jesus?"

To think on that which is lovely is to think on that which is winsome. "The Greek is *prosphiles*, and it might be paraphrased as that which calls forth love. There are those whose minds are so set on vengeance and punishment that they call forth bitterness and fear in others. There are those whose minds are so set on criticism and rebuke that they call forth resentment in others. The mind of the Christian is set on the lovely things—kindness, sympathy, forbearance—so he is a winsome person, whom to see is to love."[14]

To think on that which is admirable, or of good repute, means to think on that which is "Well–spoken of, of good report, praiseworthy, laudable."[15] When your mind struggles, you especially cannot afford to waste any mind power on anything that is degrading to yourself or others. We as believers have been given the mind of Christ, as well as mind-transforming Scripture. We have no place dwelling on the corrupt thoughts found in the world.

To think on that which is excellent is to think on that which with is pleasing to God and to think on that which is worthy of praise means that which is praiseworthy and deserving of applause.

On these types of thoughts we are to think about. While it might not come naturally, reminding ourselves often of this practical list that Paul has given us will give us a standard to align our thoughts with. If your thought does not fall into one of those categories, ask God to help you make that thought obedient to Him.

If you are struggling, let me encourage you today. There is hope, and so much of it. Even if you recognize your thoughts to be toxic or irrational, yet are frustrated that you feel enslaved to them, believe with me that nothing is too big for God to handle. A number of tools can be learned through therapy, which I believe to be a good gift from God. For instance, my therapist had to teach me how to tell the difference between a thought and a feeling. Oftentimes the tangle of thoughts and feelings can be overwhelming. But the more you learn and practice how to distinguish a thought from a feeling, The more second nature it becomes. So, let's break it down.

Thought: I feel like nobody cares.

Feeling: sad

We must learn the difference between our thoughts from our feelings. Throwing the word "feel" in the thought may trick us to believe that that string of words is our feeling, but really that one word (sad) is the feeling.

Sit in that feeling.

Feel the feeling.

It's not sinful to feel sad.

Now take that thought and compare it to the Scripture, which is the Truth we live by as children of God. "Give all your worries and cares to God, for he cares about you" (1 Peter 5:7 NLT).

According to Scripture, God cares for you. This should challenge the thought: "Nobody cares for me." Even still fully aware of the feeling of sadness radiating through your being, you can preach truth to yourself. You can remind yourself that you are fully loved and deeply cared about.

This is taking your thought captive and making it obedient to Christ. This is setting your thoughts on things above and renewing your mind with the Word of God. This is thinking about the goodness of God in your difficult circumstances, which will infuse your sorrow with joy.

And never for one second forget that Jesus understands the struggle. If you'll remember, Jesus was baptized, tempted in the desert, and then His ministry began. While in the desert, which can be found at the beginning of Luke chapter 4, satan tempted Jesus, but we see Jesus always respond with Scripture as a way to fight back with Truth.

> One practical implication we may draw from this passage is that temptation itself is not a sin. Jesus was "tempted in every way, just as we are—yet was without sin" (Heb. 4:15; see also 2 Cor. 5:21). A misunderstanding

of this defeats many people before they begin resisting temptation. A false (devilish) guilt grips them, and they begin to lose the battle before they begin to fight it. . . . It is possible to fast forty days without food, but not without water, especially in an arid, hot climate like the Judean wilderness. The understatement about Jesus' hunger is intended to show that Jesus fought his battle with a serious handicap but still came out victorious.[16]

At the beginning of the temptation, Scripture says, "Then Jesus left the Jordan, full of the Holy Spirit, and was led by the Spirit in the wilderness for forty days to be tempted by the devil" (Luke 4:1–2a CSB), and it ends by saying, "Then Jesus returned to Galilee in the power of the Spirit" (Luke 4:14).

Jesus was never without the Holy Spirit, and neither are you as a follower of Christ. The Holy Spirit fills you, leads you, gives you power, and helps you victoriously endure all temptation. We cannot look at the Holy Spirit's role in the temptation of Christ and blame God from temptation, but what we see here is that the devil has no power to act independently of God. Nothing happens to you outside the knowledge and sovereignty of God, which is a comforting place to be, given the good character of the Father.

Perhaps you cannot control whether or not the intrusive thought enters your mind, but you can control what you do with it. Mental illness may handicap your ability to think clearly, but you have a Savior who understands. The unsettling thoughts might accompany your mental illness, but you are more than a conqueror through the Most High.

You can say no to a life of settled rebellion. You can set your mind on the things above. You can be trained to look to the unseen rather than the seen. You can ask God to give you the strength to take your thoughts captive. And when you fail, you can get up and try again. Imperfect progress is still progress.

Therefore, since we have a great high priest who has passed through the heavens—Jesus the Son of God—let us hold fast to our confession. For we do not have a high priest who is unable to sympathize with our weaknesses, but one who has been tempted in every way as we are, yet without sin. Therefore, let us approach the throne of grace with boldness, so that we may receive mercy and find grace to help us in time of need.

(Hebrews 4:14–16 CSB)

Mental illness might bend your mind toward death, but the death and resurrection of Jesus means that death has no hold on you. And praise God for the provision of medication which can often help the mind to settle so that the hard yet holy work of growth in your ability to live out your faith can happen.

Rest in that grace today—God gives you everything you need to win the battle in your mind, and if you've been opposed to utilizing modern medicine, let me ask you to pray that the Lord would help you see His plan for your healing, which very well may include earthly means as He accomplishes His divine plan in and through you.

5

A Bound Daughter

Six months had passed since we moved home from Turkey, and I had been hospitalized for the second time. I was at a statewide Christian women's retreat alongside thousands of other women.

I was a Christian.

I was a woman.

I was learning from some of the most well-known teachers of the day.

I loved the girl time.

You'd think I'd be having the time of my life .

But I felt 100 percent out of place and completely broken inside.

Everything was beautiful from the setting to the joy that I saw radiate from those around me. One really can be lonely even while surrounded by people. I questioned if I still believed the words they were singing with their eyes closed and hands raised.

Only months prior I was serving the Lord overseas with a great sense of purpose, but there I stood in a completely different context, culture, and on a different continent. My fall felt great, and I was having a difficult time processing everything.

Only a few friends knew the war raging in my mind and the recent hospitalizations I lived through. If any other lady there knew what it was like to live with mental illness, I sure didn't know, and like many of them, hiding the torment in my mind for eighteen years was how I knew to survive and fit in. As is typically more socially acceptable, I smiled on the outside all the while feeling completely alone in the secret places of my heart. My doctor and my therapist were treating me, and while my understanding of mental illness, as well as my ability to cope were both improving, when in a church setting, I still felt awkward and ashamed. Six whole months of pursuing mental health after my breakdown in Turkey, and shame still held my hand tight.

The enemy loves to convince us that no one else struggles like we do. Satan's plans thrive when he can deceive us to believe that we are alone or that our struggles are worse than everyone else's. I'm learning that sometimes it only takes one person to start an entire movement of authenticity. And true community blossoms where there is vulnerability. We must never assume that no one else can understand our struggles since "No temptation has come upon you except what is common to humanity" (1 Corinthians 10:13 CSB).

As bedtime approached, I hid in my bottom bunk bed to discreetly swallow the medicine I was new to taking and still felt shame and disgust over. I picked up my pill box and dropped it right away. My hands shook. Pills scattered all over the tile floor. Women looked as I scrambled desperately to pick them up. Each bounce they made sounded as if it were playing through a megaphone. The thought of being found out and labeled "mentally ill" was so mortifying to me that I felt frantic with anxiety as I sat there with no way to reverse all that just happened.

Two girls came to my rescue as another one of my friends came over to me and asked if I needed to talk. I loved her, trusted her, and sadly, in a moment of panic, lashed out at her. I stormed past her and went outside where I cried. Not exactly the picture of a woman who knew how to pull herself together in a healthy way or who was enjoying herself. I was trying to survive, and I felt trapped in the middle of wanting to fit in. But instead, felt broken compared to others.

While sitting in that bunk bed, I never would have imagined that I would someday not only be in women's ministry, voluntarily speaking out about mental illness, but I would be asked to speak on that very stage in Oklahoma, in that very room where I felt so out of place. But that's the redemption of God. He uses our brokenness to uniquely gift us with compassion for others.

Before the victory of grasping the purpose in my pain, came the days of enduring and continuing to show up to church despite the awkwardness I felt or the moments where I came undone. It was actually during this season of enduring that I found myself in a Sunday school class where we were studying the book of Luke.

It was right there in that room, tucked away in my home church, that I would have an encounter with God that would leave me changed forever. We read about an unnamed woman in Scripture who I believe could relate to feeling alone or like all eyes were on her, and as we read her story, my heart softened to receive God's Word.

The book of Luke was written "So that his readers would understand that the gospel is for all, both Jews and Gentiles alike, since Jesus is the promised one of God as prophesied in the OT and as attested through God's saving activity in Jesus' life, death, and resurrection."[1]

> The events in the book of Luke take place almost entirely within the vicinity of Palestine, an area extending roughly from Caesarea Philippi in the north

to Beersheba in the south. During this time it was ruled by the Roman Empire. The opening chapters describe the events surrounding Jesus' birth in Judea, where Herod had been appointed king by the Romans. The closing chapters end with Jesus' death, resurrection, and ascension during the rule of Pontius Pilate and the tetrarchs Antipas and Philip.[2]

Luke depicts Jesus in his ministry as deeply compassionate and we really see this in the story of the woman. Our entire story takes place in the synagogue. Although opposition was on the rise from the religious leaders, Jesus was still welcome in synagogues. The Greek word synagogue simply means "assembly," and was the place where Jews would gather for instruction and worship in the New Testament period. You could think of this as a church in our culture today. The size of the synagogue varied with the population of the area, and the building was designed so that the worshipers, as they entered for prayers, the reading of Scripture and a sermon explaining the Scripture, looked toward Jerusalem. As seen in Scripture, Jesus could be found in synagogues, both teaching and healing in them.

Jesus was an adult when his ministry began. After His baptism and temptation in the desert, we see Jesus begin His ministry in a synagogue were he stood up to read.

> And the scroll of the prophet Isaiah was given to him. He unrolled the scroll and found the place where it was written, 'The Spirit of the Lord is upon me, because he has anointed me to proclaim good news to the poor. He has sent me to proclaim liberty to the captives and covering of sight to the blind, to set at liberty those who are oppressed, to proclaim the year of the Lord's favor.' "
> (Luke 4:17–19 ESV).

We also find Jesus in the synagogue for the setting of our story about the unnamed woman, but this time it will be the last record of Him in a synagogue. "Now he was teaching in one of the synagogues on the Sabbath. And behold, there was a woman who had had a disabling spirit for eighteen years. She was bent over and could not fully straighten herself" (Luke 13:10–11 ESV).

Let's step back a moment and imagine the scene. She was a woman who was physically bent over because of a "disabling spirit," or a "spirit of infirmity" as some translations put it. The word "disabling" in verse 11 is the Greek word *asthenia*. This word means weakness, sickness, and disease. "That evil spirits or demons can cause such bodily weakness is evident from Luke 13:11. In this passage the woman is probably suffering physical results of a spiritual or attitudinal cause, such a disease being psychosomatic, as we say today."[3]

The term *psychosomatic* means "of, relating to, involving, or concerned with bodily symptoms caused by mental or emotional disturbance" (Merriam-Webster). This woman was in distress, both mentally and physically, evidently having a spinal problem, which left her in a crippling state for eighteen years. "Demonic activity seemed to be responsible for her chronic and lengthy disease, although Luke does not say that the woman was demon possessed."[4] Because her condition was called a "disabling spirit," or a "spirit of infirmity," we can see that her physical malady was linked with her spiritual condition.

> The physical condition of the woman was pitiable in the extreme. For eighteen long years she had endured her deformity, described first of all as "a spirit of infirmity" which does not mean that she was of a weak and infirm spirit. The phrase denotes one of those mysterious derangements of the nervous system, having the rise in the mind rather in the body. Her physical curvature was a consequence of mental obliquity, making her melancholy. Thus her strange malady was partly physical and partly mental.[5]

Like Paul, who could not rid himself of the "messenger of Satan" that God gave him in 2 Corinthians 12, I wonder if she ever begged God to remove this thorn in her flesh. Eighteen years is an excruciatingly long time to endure affliction. Had she adopted David's cry found in Psalm 13:1–3 (CSB) as her own heart's cry? "How long, Lord? Will you forget me forever? How long will you hide your face from me? How long will I store up anxious concerns within me, agony in my mind every day? How long will my enemy dominate me? Consider me and answer, Lord my God. Restore brightness to my eyes; otherwise, I will sleep in death." Like David in Psalm 56:8 (NLT) I imagine her saying to God "You keep track of all my sorrows. You have collected all my tears in your bottle."

God hears your cries too. Each and every sorrow of your heart and mind does not go unnoticed by the Lord. Each tear that has stained your pillow has been collected in His bottle. Each physical pain, regardless of its origin, is seen by the God Who Sees. If you are in a place of agony where you cannot fix yourself, please know that the woman was the same.

We are told in the text that she could not straighten herself. She was completely incapable of making herself well. Have you ever been told to just shake it off or choose to be happy when it comes to mental illness? A common misconception is that those with mental illness can make themselves get better though sheer determination, but that's not true. Like that woman, I understand what it feels like to be so downcast that I cannot straighten myself.

We don't know whether or not she cried out to God for healing, but we do know that she didn't allow her bowed down posture keep her from being in the synagogue on that day. This beautiful detail suggests her faithfulness to attending despite her condition. She was there among the healthy even though as a woman of such humble appearance, she would have certainly felt the forced humility that came with such lowly a position in society.

Like I felt out of place at the women's retreat, among other believers worshiping, praying, and studying Scripture, I wonder if she did too. Regardless of how she felt, she still did the next right thing. She didn't allow the shame of her appearance or the torment of being bound by satan keep her isolated at home. No, she showed up. She kept doing the very next thing as she endured. And we can show up too.

Charles Spurgeon's insight on this woman is powerful and applicable:

> Our Lord was in the synagogue, and there was she. She might very well have said, "It is very painful for me to go into a public place; I ought to be excused." But no, there she was. Dear child of God, the devil has sometimes suggested to you that it is vain for you to go any more to hear the word. Go all the same. He knows you are likely to escape from his hands so long as you hear the word, and therefore if he can keep you away he will do so. It was while in the house of prayer that this woman found her liberty, and there you may find it; therefore still continue to go up to the house of the Lord, come what may.[6]

So we have our woman, crippled into an extremely downcast posture, tormented from being bound by satan, and quietly among the others listening to Jesus. Perhaps she was a regular worshiper in the synagogue since no one took special note of her. No one until Jesus that is. "When Jesus saw her, he called her over and said to her, 'Woman, you are freed from your disability.' And he laid his hands on her, and immediately she was made straight, and she glorified God" (Luke 13:12–13 ESV).

Satan may have bound her to where her face was looking down into her grave, but he could not force her into it. God's plan would prevail. This woman so bent over possibly could not even see Jesus, but regardless, Jesus saw her. He saw her and He called her. He is the one who initiated. Jesus sees you too, dear one. Maybe you feel invisible or ashamed, lonely or humiliated by your circumstance.

Know that Jesus sees you and He is the one who calls you to Himself. Jesus is the one who took the initiative in this story of healing, for aside from being present at the synagogue, she exhibited no faith or attempt to find healing. Like others in Scripture who sought out Jesus and went to extreme measures to be near Him, this woman's story is different. She was simply present, and she was herself. Jesus did not require her to tidy up her life or help herself before He would help her, and this shows the beautiful compassion of Christ. Whoever coined the phrase "God helps those who help themselves" perhaps needs to take a look at this woman. God loves you exactly as you are but He also loves you too much to leave you exactly as you are.

If you feel Jesus calling you to Himself, don't let your physical, emotional, spiritual, or mental state keep you from obeying like the woman. When Jesus laid His hands on her, she was immediately healed. As her spine straightened, and the invisible chains satan bound her in were broken she experienced complete and lasting healing. It wasn't her attendance to a religious service or activity that saved her, but rather it was a personal experience with Jesus that broke the bond of satan over her mind and body. So it is with us. Church is good, but it's Jesus Himself that transforms.

Perhaps, like this woman, you haven't given up on church yet, but find yourself bent over spiritually with no ability to change. Maybe your needs have felt too overwhelming to have hope of change and you have been overlooked by others around you. Remember, "No creature is hidden from his sight, but all are naked and exposed to the eyes of him whom we must give account" (Hebrew 4:13 ESV), and no darkness you struggle with is too much for God, for you can look to Him and say with confidence: "Even the darkness is not dark to you; the night is bright as the day, for darkness is as light with you" (Psalm 139:12 ESV).

While her healing is definitely worth our notice, so is her beautiful response to the healing. The Bible says her immediate response was glorifying God. We don't see her give into bitterness for the eighteen years she was bound, and we don't see her get angry that God allowed satan to bind her. No, her immediate reaction was thankfulness. It was praise! The imperfect tense of the word "glorify" (Greek: *doxazo*), shows that she was giving glory to God over and over and again and again. Can you say the same for you? This response is birthed from a heart that sees God as sovereign and worthy of our trust.

We may not understand why things happen, and we may never understand this side of heaven, but we can endure with hope that our God is always working for our good and for His glory. Like Psalm 107:20–21 (NLT) may our hearts sing

> He sent out his word and healed them,
>   snatching them from the door of death.
> Let them praise the LORD for his great love
>   and for the woderful things he has done for them.

Our story, however, does not end there with her praise, for "the ruler of the synagogue, indignant because Jesus had healed on the Sabbath, said to the people, 'There are six days in which work ought to be done. Come on those days and be healed, and not on the Sabbath day'" (Luke 13:14 ESV). "Because Jesus had healed on the Sabbath, the ruler's indignation was aroused, completely ignoring the woman's being freed from 18 years of suffering. Jesus was not violating any OT commandment; later Jewish traditions had added many more commandments and prohibitions that God had ever given his Word."[7]

In response to the ruler of the synagogue, "the Lord answered him, 'You hypocrites! Does not each of you on the Sabbath untie his ox or his donkey from the manger and lead it away to water it?'" (Luke 13:15 ESV). Through His question, Jesus showed the hypocrisy of those who would elevate ritualistic observations over human beings, thus humiliating the leader rather than Jesus.

This is just who Jesus is. He is about people and relationships. He is about compassion and healing. He loves and sees those in need of a Savior, and He calls them to Himself. But He doesn't stop there. He continued, "'and ought not this woman, a daughter of Abraham whom Satan bound for eighteen years, be loosed from this bond on the Sabbath day?' As he said these things, all his adversaries were put to shame, and all the people rejoiced at all the glorious things that were done by him" (Luke 13:16–27 ESV).

Included in this story is a precious treasure we cannot overlook. Jesus called the newly freed woman a "daughter of Abraham." He called her by her identity. He didn't refer to anything regarding her behavior, appearance, or the eighteen long years she spent in satan's bondage.

No, He called her by her belief. Did you know that as a follower of Christ, you are also a child of Abraham through your faith? Abraham is known for many things in the Bible, but the thing that set him apart was his faith. "For what does the Scripture say? Abraham believed God, and it was credited to him for righteousness" (Romans 4:3 CSB). "You know, then, that those who have faith, these are Abraham's sons. Now the Scripture saw in advance that God would justify the Gentiles by faith and proclaimed the gospel ahead of time to Abraham, saying, All the nations will be blessed through you. Consequently, those who have faith are blessed with Abraham, who had faith" (Galatians 3:7–9 CSB).

She was a daughter of Abraham, and so are you as a child of God, but your identity doesn't stop there. One of satan's most effective weapons against Christians are the lies he tempts us to believe about who we are and whose we are.

But something happens when a child of God starts replacing lies with Truth. The Truth sets them free; joy penetrates their sorrow; and thriving in the midst of mental illness becomes possible. Perhaps the lies still burn as fiery darts from the enemy, but like those of faith mentioned in Hebrews 11:34 (CSB), may it be said of you, too, that you "gained strength in weakness, became mighty in battle, and put foreign armies to flight." The more you practice telling yourself the truth of who you are and Who you belong to, the mightier you become in battle.

Mental Illness tells you:

- You are unwanted.
- You don't belong.
- You are worthless.
- There is not hope for your life.
- You are broken.
- You can't win against evil.
- How you treat your body doesn't matter.
- Your ministry is over.
- You are a burden.

God tells you:

- You are His child (John 1:12).
- You are Christ's friend (John 15:15).
- You have been bought with a price and belong to God (1 Corinthians 6:19–20).
- God will finish the work He started in you (Philippians 1:6).
- You are complete in Christ (Colossians 2:10).

- You are born of God and evil cannot touch you (1 John 5:18).
- You are God's temple (1 Corinthians 3:16).
- You have been appointed to bear fruit (John 15:16).
- You can approach God with freedom and confidence (Ephesians 3:12).

You are a child of Abraham, and ultimately a child of God. Maybe you're still bound by mental illness, but just keep doing the next right thing while you trust and wait and hope and believe. Jesus sees you and the mental illness you are living with is not a character flaw. Perhaps others have lead you to believe that you are suffering because of your own foolish choices, but that is not always the case with mental illness.

Unlike other healing stories in the gospels, there is no mention of this woman's sin being the reason for her disability. Her first response is also one of praise and publicly and immediately glorifying God. Here we are, thousands of years later, being encouraged by this woman's perseverance and healing. Imagine if she would have chosen to succumb to satan's plan for her, by giving up and isolating herself at home.

Another story comes to my mind where we see Jesus heal a man with a disability. "As he was passing by, he saw a man blind from birth. His disciples asked him, 'Rabbi, who sinned, this man or his parents, that he was born blind?' 'Neither this man nor his parents sinned,' Jesus answered. This came about so that God's works might be displayed in him" (John 9:1–3 CSB).

In this story, we again see the sovereignty of God in the disabilities of people. Even the disciples assumed sin was the reason behind the man's blindness, but Jesus said that the reason he was born blind was so that the glory of God could be shown through his healing.

The Bible does trace suffering to moral causes. For example, death came ultimately to all because of Adam's sin (Romans 5:12–21). Children do sometimes suffer because of the sins of their parents (Exodus 34:7). One of the greatest tragedies of sin comes in its far-reaching effect, hurting the innocent as well as the guilty. Personal sin can also cause suffering (Deuteronomy 28:15–68; Jeremiah 31:30). However, biblical teachings have been distorted and misunderstood. Jesus replied clearly that in this case the man's blindness had been allowed so that God's works might be displayed in him. What a comforting blessing to know that in suffering one can exalt Christ (Romans 8:28; 1 Peter 2:21).[8]

If you find yourself suffering today, may you look to your God and with great confidence say, "The LORD opens the eyes of the blind. The LORD lifts up those who are weighed down. The LORD loves the godly" (Psalm 146:8 NLT).

There is a reason for your circumstances far beyond what we can see, but God can and will bring good from any evil meant to harm you. It's just who He is.

6

Mentally Ill
for God's Glory

I sit at my favorite writing spot in my kitchen in Oklahoma at 5:30 in the morning. I'm holding in my hands an old leather journal that I started writing in as a new follower of Jesus in 2004. I flip through my journal and can see a progression.

My entries began quite shallow and remain that way until 2012. This is the year after my dad's death and the year I see a large shift in my journal. There is a sudden downward spiral in the mood of my words as darkness and pain are woven throughout the rest of my journal's pages. I can see that I was simply quoting verses and singing praises of God in my journal in the beginning, but following the trauma of being abandoned by my dad, I started deepening in my understanding of what it means to be real with God.

It's as though I was afraid to have any questions or struggles prior to being left by my dad. But this is the beauty of endurance. And not just gritting your teeth and bearing it, for the idea of enduring in the Bible has a much richer meaning. Endurance (*hupomone*) means to abide under.

> The root idea of hupomone is to remain under some discipline, subjecting one's self to something against

which demands the submission of one's will to something against which one naturally would rebel. It portrays a picture of steadfastly and unflinchingly bearing up under a heavy load and describes that quality of character which does not allow one to surrender to circumstances or succumb under trial. . . .

. . . Hupomone does not describe a grim resignation or a passive "grin and bear" attitude but a triumphant facing of difficult circumstances knowing that even out of evil God guarantees good. It is courageous gallantry which accepts suffering and hardship and turns them into grace and glory. For believers, it is a steadfastness, especially as God enables us to "remain under" (or endure) whatever challenges, trials, tests, afflictions, etc, He providentially allows in our life.[1]

There will come a time when you look back at the past and see the goodness of God in how He has refined you in your endurance. In that shift in my journal, I can see that my relationship was growing with my heavenly Father, and it was really just the beginning of a beautiful life as His daughter.

One of the earliest entries where I can finally see I'm starting to grow is in a journal entry dated November 8, 2012, in which I quoted Oswald Chambers.

At times God puts us through the discipline of darkness to teach us to heed Him. Song birds are taught to sing in the dark, and we are put into the shadow of God's hand until we learn to hear Him. "What I tell you in darkness"—watch where God puts you into darkness, and when you are there keep your mouth shut. Are you in the dark just now in your circumstances, or in your life with God? Then remain quiet. If you open your mouth in the dark, you will talk in the wrong mood: darkness is the time to listen. Don't talk to other people about it; don't read books to find out the reason of the darkness, but listen and heed. If you talk to other people, you cannot hear what God is saying. When you

are in the dark, listen, and God will give you a very
precious message for someone else when you get into
the light.[2]

As I read thoughtfully over each word in my own
handwriting, I thought back to those days as a newly orphaned
young adult trying to navigate my twenties. I think back to
just how much loss and pain and darkness would still be in
the years ahead of me and my heart drops. But most of all I
wish more than anything that I could take my sweet, young
face in my hands and tell myself that someday this will make
more sense, and that while my dad choosing to abandon me
through death would leave a gaping hole in my heart tainted
with deeply believed lies that I was unlovable, someday God
would convince me of His deep, abiding love. So much so
that I would be given the platform to share this message with
others. With you.

So here I am, obeying Jesus who once said "What I tell you
in the dark, speak in the light. What you hear in a whisper,
proclaim on the housetops" (Matthew 10:27 CSB). Many
years of quiet growth with God took place before I was ever
ready to share publicly about mental illness and suffering. But
when the time came to proclaim to from the rooftops all that
He whispered in the decades of darkness, I have truly come to
a point where thankfulness for the trials runs deep.

The freedom I feel today is akin to resurrection from the
dead. In the dark early days of finally pursuing mental health,
God illuminated the story of Lazarus, helping me understand
that I am loved even though I am allowed to be sick.

When God convinces you of His love, no wound or wall or
anything else in your heart can hold Him back. When people
would tell me they loved me, those precious words seemed to
bounce off my numb heart and mind as a bouncy ball on the
kitchen floor, that is until the Lord intervened.

Embracing the Lord's love was an essential step on my journey toward mental health and as you read this story of Lazarus, allow these words from the mouth of God to hold you tightly and speak tenderly to your hurting heart: "Do not fear, for I have redeemed you; I have called you by your name; you are mine" (Isaiah 43:1 CSB). As a redeemed Child of God, you are called by name and you belong to the God who is love. May that identity sink down deep in your soul and be at the forefront of your mind as you continue reading.

"Now a man was sick, Lazarus from Bethany, the village of Mary and her sister Martha. Mary was the one who anointed the Lord with perfume and wiped his feet with her hair, and it was her brother Lazarus who was sick. So the sisters sent a message to him: 'Lord, the one you love is sick'" (John 11:1–3 CSB).

While I read this story in the gospel of John, verse 3 struck me deeply, causing me to pause and ponder. If the Lord loved the man named Lazarus, why would He allow sickness to consume his body? My natural inclination toward my children, whom I love, is to try and protect them from anything and everything that might inflict sickness on their bodies or pain in their hearts. So why would God, who is good in every way, and loves His children with perfect, infinite love, allow His loved one to fall sick?

> It is no new thing for those whom Christ loves, to be sick; bodily distempers correct the corruption, and try the graces of God's people. He came not to preserve his people from these afflictions, but to save them from their sins, and from the wrath to come; however, it behooves us to apply to Him in behalf of our friends and relatives when sick and afflicted. Let this reconcile us to the darkest dealings of Providence, that they are all for the glory of God: sickness, loss, disappointment, are so; and if God be glorified, we ought to be satisfied.[3]

While barely tiptoeing into this beloved story, my eyes were violently ripped open as I was inevitably being forced to address the question that was layered deep down in my heart: "If God loves me, why does He let me have mental illness?" With that question in mind, I continued reading.

"When Jesus heard it, he said, 'This sickness will not end in death but is for the glory of God, so that the Son of God may be glorified through it'" (John 11:4 CSB). Jesus did not hesitate in comforting his loved ones by giving them a glimpse into the plan and purposes of God. "This sickness is not unto death—The word 'death' here is equivalent to remaining under death, Romans 6:23. 'The wages of sin is death'—permanent or unchanging death, opposed to eternal life. Jesus evidently did not intend to deny that he would die. The words which he immediately adds show that he would expire, and that he would raise him up to show forth the power and glory of God."[4]

"Now Jesus loved Martha and her sister and Lazarus. So when he heard that Lazarus was sick, he stayed where he was two more days, and then he said to the disciples, 'Let's go back to Judea'" (John 11:5–7). While reading those next words of the story, my mind zeroed in on verse 6: "So when he heard that Lazarus was sick, he stayed where he was two more days."

If Jesus loved Martha, her sister, and Lazarus, then why would He voluntarily stay two more days? Why would He delay? By choosing the wait, the sisters were forced to experience the agony of watching their beloved die, and Lazarus went through the horror of actually feeling his body shut down. Yes, the power of Jesus would be beautifully demonstrated, but these people, who were precious to Jesus, needed to suffer first.

Why? Because Jesus loved them.

For what purpose? The glory of God.

That seems completely counterintuitive in our finite thinking.

Jesus loved them so much that He allowed them to walk through the valley of the shadow of death, but as the Good Shepherd that He is, He didn't let the story end there. And considering that Jesus being glorified was the main goal, I was confronted with an idea that can be hard to grasp when my mind struggles, and I tend to turn inward in pain: It's not all about me.

Jesus acted in a way that didn't make sense to them, but He knew it was for the growth of their faith and the displaying of His glory. The Lord loved them too much to act like they expected, and He won't be bound by human logic. When our human minds cannot wrap themselves around the way God works, it can lead to distrust and ultimately unbelief, which is dangerous territory because as the Word says, it is impossible to please God without faith (Hebrews 11:6).

The love of Christ is so unfathomable that we must depend on Spirit-wrought strength to understand, because without the Spirit, His love can be confusing. We also must not forget about the Helper, or the Holy Spirit, whom Jesus said, "the Father will send in my name, he will teach you all things and bring to your remembrance all that I have said to you" (John 14:26 ESV). We understand the sometimes confusing love of God when we do so through the power of the Holy Spirit.

But I really do get what you might be thinking right now. Jesus is compassionate, so doesn't He see how I suffer with depression and want to heal me? Can't Jesus rid my mind and body of the effects of trauma if He really is the Prince of Peace? Yes, yes, He can. But what we find in this story is that the love of Christ waits, and it's in the waiting that our faith is forged and shines with the glory of the God who is always working for your good.

Perhaps you're waiting right now, but you are not alone in mourning over the way you are being forced to wait on God's timing. It was David who lamented, "How long, Lord?

Will you forget me forever? How long will you hide your face from me? How long will I store up anxious concerns within me, agony in my mind every day? How long will my enemy dominate me?" (Psalm 13:1–2 CSB). David was not sinning by his expression of weariness, but rather crying out to a God he believed to be good and capable of handling his frustration and questions.

Regarding the sometimes confusing ways of God,

> Beyond all doubt this was just to let things come to their worst, in order to display His glory. But how trying, meantime, to the faith of his friends, and how unlike the way in which love to a dying friend usually shows itself, on which it is plain that Mary reckoned. But the ways of divine are not as the ways of human love. Often they are the reverse. When His people are sick, in body or spirit; when their case is waxing more and more desperate every day; when all hope of recovery is about to expire—just then and therefore it is that "He abides two days still in the same place where He is." Can they still hope against hope? Often they do not; but "this is their infirmity." For it is His chosen style of acting.[5]

We must remember that when God acts unpredictably, it comes from His great love and knowledge that His plan is perfect. It will all make sense one day. He sees the whole picture while we see just a tiny glimpse and our emotions can often even cloud that small view. When God's behavior does not align with what we think it should be, we must stand firm on who He is. When we remember that He is good, loving, merciful, full of light, and always for us, we can look at His unpredictably through eyes of faith and hearts of hope.

> He said to the disciples, "Let's go to Judea again."
> "Rabbi," the disciples told him, "just now the Jews tried to stone you, and you're going there again?"
> "Aren't there twelve hours in a day?" Jesus answered.

"If anyone walks during the day, he doesn't stumble, because he sees the light of this world. But if anyone walks during the night, he does stumble, because the light is not in him."

He said this, and then he told them, "Our friend Lazarus has fallen asleep, but I'm on my way to wake him up."

Then the disciples said to him, "Lord, if he has fallen asleep, he will get well."

Jesus, however, was speaking about his death, but they thought he was speaking about natural sleep. So Jesus then told them plainly, "Lazarus has died. I'm glad for you that I wasn't there so that you may believe. But let's go to him." (John 11:7–15 CSB)

To the disciples, the thought of going back to the place where the Jews tried to kill Jesus was frightening and unreasonable. This is how the human mind works. When trauma happens, hypervigilance takes up residence, for to be human is to have the propensity for self-preservation and the inclination to protect yourself and your loved ones from danger.

Their question did make sense with human logic, but we must remember that God is far above us. His ways will never be our ways and His understanding of what is good and loving for us will always be perfect, regardless of whether or not it makes sense at the time. God does not make decisions from a place of hypervigilance, which is so very comforting.

Jesus, who feels emotion just like you and I do, can look at any situation from a perspective that sees the entire picture, for He does not ever experience emotional hijacking. We must remember this when our thoughts carry us off into anxiety. This tension of anxiously seeing our circumstance as one way, but knowing that God is in control, is where trust is born in His children.

Suffering offers a uniquely beautiful opportunity to look at God and say, "I don't understand, but I know You do, and I will trust You." In Psalm 13, David may have openly complained before the Lord, asking Him "How long, Lord? Will you forget me forever? How long will you hide your face from me? How long will I store up anxious concerns within me, agony in my mind every day? How long will my enemy dominate me?" (Psalm 13:1–2 CSB).

But His lament did not stop there. As a lament is meant to do, David was brought to a place of hope and trust when he ended his cry to God by saying, "But I have trusted in your faithful love; my heart will rejoice in your deliverance. I will sing to the Lord because he has treated me generously," (Psalm 13:5–6 CSB). Did his feelings of anguish suddenly subside? Probably not. Was he preaching truth to Himself and therefore able to continue on in life? Absolutely.

And so, Jesus did go to the scene of His friend's death, but not in the timing that makes sense to us. "When Jesus arrived, he found that Lazarus had already been in the tomb four days. Bethany was near Jerusalem (less than two miles away). Many of the Jews had come to Martha and Mary to comfort them about their brother" (John 11:17–19 CSB).

> Burial usually took place the day of death because of the hot climate and lack of knowledge about preserving the body. The body would be prepared for burial by anointing with special and expensive spices and ointments and then by wrapping the body in strips of white cloth. Jesus did not begin His journey from across the Jordan until a day or two after Lazarus died, which, together with a journey of several days to reach Judea, meant that He did not arrive until four days after Lazarus's burial. Jewish tradition claimed that the soul hovered over the body three days, in hope of a reunion, until decomposition of the body began to be evident. However superstitious and untrue, the widespread acceptance of this idea may have played into Jesus' timing of His arrival in Bethany. No Jew could doubt

that the resurrection of Lazarus from the grave after four days was indeed a miracle.[6]

What an agonizing four days that must have been for the sisters of Lazarus. "As soon as Martha heard that Jesus was coming, she went to meet him, but Mary remained seated in the house. Then Martha said to Jesus, 'Lord, if you had been here, my brother wouldn't have died. Yet even now I know that whatever you ask from God, God will give you'" (John 11:20–22 CSB).

My heart resonates deeply with Mary here in the story. Have you ever looked at a loss in your life and said something like, "God if you would have done something or been there for me, then this wouldn't have happened." While Martha's statement to Christ includes a mild rebuke, we still see her faith in acknowledging that God would give Jesus whatever He asked Him for.

She questions, but she didn't give up. May this be our heart as well when trying to make sense of God's allowance of something as difficult as mental illness. This is a beautiful picture that shows where our human understanding and our faith intersect.

The first part of her statement was the human reaction, but as her faith took over, she was able to declare the truth that Jesus could ask God and receive from Him. When things don't turn out at as we think they ought to have, we can be like Martha and look backward.

But Jesus, as He always does, points her to the future. And when our vision is facing forward, expectation fills our heart with hope. Don't look back at what you think should have been, but look forward, for this forward-facing gaze invites joy into our present sorrow. We cannot forget as we continue on in this story that it began with the declaration that Jesus loved those who were experiencing loss and that because He loved them so, He waited and allowed the suffering to take place.

Every single thing that happens to you, whether it be the diagnosis of mental illness, or even the suicide of a loved one where God allowed them to die, must be mourned from a place that is settled in the fact that God loves you. It may not ever make sense in our human minds on this earth, but we can hold fast to that as a fact that remains regardless of how dire our situation may seem.

God is love. He acts from a place of love. He holds back at times from a heart of love. He allows tragedy because of His love. "No, in all these things we are more than conquerors through him who loved us. For I am persuaded that neither death nor life, nor angels nor rulers, nor things present nor things to come, nor powers, nor height nor depth, nor any other created thing will be able to separate us from the love of God that is in Christ Jesus our Lord" (Romans 8:37–39 CSB). He will never stop loving you and nothing, not even mental illness or suicide can separate you from this perfect love.

In the story, in response to Martha, we see Jesus say,

> "Your brother will rise again," Jesus told her.
> Martha said to him, "I know that he will rise again in the resurrection at the last day."
> Jesus said to her, "I am the resurrection and the life. The one who believes in me, even if he dies, will live. Everyone who lives and believes in me will never die. Do you believe this?"
> "Yes, Lord," she told him, "I believe you are the Messiah, the Son of God, who comes into the world."
> (John 11:23–27 CSB)

We see in Martha's words, an affirmation of end-time resurrection that certainly was in line with the beliefs of the Pharisees, the majority of the Jews, as well as even the teaching of Jesus. But Martha misunderstood the fullness of Jesus's promise. I love what Jesus does here in our story: He takes the belief Martha already expressed in resurrection and directs it at Himself.

"Jesus does not merely say that he will bring about the resurrection or that he will be the cause of the resurrection (both of which are true), but something much stronger: I am the resurrection. Resurrection from the dead and genuine eternal life in fellowship with God are so closely tied to Jesus that they're embodied in him and can be found only in relationship with him. Therefore believes in me implies personal trust in Christ."[7]

> Having said this, she went back and called her sister Mary, saying in private, "The Teacher is here and is calling for you."
> As soon as Mary heard this, she got up quickly and went to him. . . . The Jews who were with her in the house consoling her saw that Mary got up quickly and went out. They followed her, supposing that she was going to the tomb to cry there.
> As soon as Mary came to where Jesus was and saw him, she fell at his feet and told him, "Lord, if you had been here, my brother wouldn't have died!"
> (John 11:28–32 CSB)

The way that Mary and Martha reacted to Christ shows their security in their relationship with Him. They knew they could be honest with Him, and I hope you know that as a child of God, you can be honest too. Martha and Mary did not attempt to hide their feelings or push them down and ignore them, but rather chose transparency with Jesus which in turn nurtured their security in Him by the way He accepted them completely as they were.

He was able to handle their confusion and questions, and He can handle yours as well. The pain they felt was real and ran deep, but the sovereignty of God allowed their genuine need to go unmet temporarily because it led to a strengthened faith which is absolutely essential in true discipleship. We see through this trial that Martha and Mary gained that maturity in faith that often comes through extreme suffering.

Jesus allowed suffering, but it was not without true compassion, and definitely not without purpose.

"When Jesus saw her crying, and the Jews who had come with her crying, he was deeply moved in his spirit and troubled. 'Where have you put him?' he asked. 'Lord,' they told him, 'come and see.' Jesus wept" (John 11:33–35 CSB).

What a profound statement that displays that humanity of Christ. He wept. This verse may be short in length, but infinitely deep in meaning. Not only was He shedding tears over His beloved friend's death, as well as for Martha and Mary who were deep in grief, but He was moved emotionally and troubled, or rather angered, by death itself as a result of sin.

But if Jesus knew the miracle of resurrection that was about to take place, then why would He cry? Jesus weeps because Lazarus experienced the darkness of death. Though Lazarus be brought forth from death, he still experienced death, and death is terrible. Jesus's reaction to death shows us that we shouldn't neglect the fact that there is a dark and evil tyranny in death. Perhaps you've lost a loved one too.

Yes, if they were a child of God, we believe they are with Jesus. Yes, it's right to believe that they will rise again, for we do not grieve without hope. But we absolutely still grieve. We can look at Jesus and see that if He wept when His friend died, all the while knowing he wouldn't stay dead long, it's OK and expected that we grieve our loved ones too. "Jesus joins his friends' sadness with heartfelt sorrow, yet underlying it is the knowledge that resurrection joy will soon follow. Jesus' example shows that heartfelt mourning in the face of death does not indicate lack of faith but honest sorrow at the reality of suffering and death."[8]

When we stop and savor the tears shed by our Savior, we see the great hope in each drop that trickled down His cheek. He understands our tears and also will one day be the one to wipe the last tear away when all things are made new. Before the joy, came the sorrow. Before the resurrection, came the death. Before the precious moment when life entered the dead body of Lazarus, came the tears.

God has a plan and is always working even now in your pain. But this moment of weeping isn't the end of our story.

> So the Jews said, "See how he loved him!" But some of them said, "Couldn't he who opened the blind man's eyes also have kept this man from dying?"
>
> Then Jesus, deeply moved again, came to the tomb. It was a cave, and a stone was lying against it. "Remove the stone," Jesus said.
>
> Martha, the dead man's sister, told him, "Lord, there is already a stench because he has been dead four days."
>
> Jesus said to her, "Didn't I tell you that if you believed you would see the glory of God?"
>
> So they removed the stone. Then Jesus raised his eyes and said, "Father, I thank you that you heard me. I know that you always hear me, but because of the crowd standing here I said this, so that they may believe you sent me." After he said this, he shouted with a loud voice, "Lazarus, come out!" The dead man came out bound hand and foot with linen strips and with his face wrapped in a cloth. Jesus said to them, "Unwrap him and let him go." (John 11:36–44 CSB)

Again, we see the love of Jesus in the way He called forth Lazarus and brought him from death to life. The love of Christ in this story allows sickness, waits for the perfect timing, weeps, but it doesn't end there, it acts; it resurrects. This radical love may challenge our small view of love, but it is at the core of this entire miracle story. But all this love that was seen in

His waiting and weeping, and even in the way He broke the bondage of death over Lazarus is meant to point to the fact that Jesus is the resurrection and life.

Jesus said: "Whoever believes in me, though he die, yet shall he live, and everyone who lives and believes in me shall never die. Do you believe this?" (John 11:25–26 ESV) This is where he was taking Martha the entire time. He's asking her if she believes His statement, even while her brother lay dead in a tomb and even tough Jesus could have prevented it from ever happening.

Jesus loved Mary, Martha, and Lazarus, and He loves you too. But because He loves you, He may wait in healing you. Love is not giving us what we want, but rather what we need. And if a life of mental illness creates in your dependency on God, a faith that moves mountains, and an unshakable hope that steadies you in the storms of life, then it is a loving thing God has given you. You may be taken through unimaginable loss and suffering in this life, but we must remember that if He delays in healing you, it's because of His great love for you. Wait and weep, but not without hope. And if the illness in your mind makes it difficult to feel loved, preach His love to yourself anyway. His love can not only resurrect the dead but can penetrate even the most broken of minds.

> When I think of all this, I fall to my knees and pray to the Father, the Creator of everything in heaven and on earth. I pray that from his glorious, unlimited resources he will empower you with inner strength through his Spirit. Then Christ will make his home in your hearts as you trust in him. Your roots will grow down into God's love and keep you strong. And may you have the power to understand, as all God's people should, how wide, how long, how high, and how deep his love is. May you experience the love of Christ, though it is too great to understand fully. Then you will be made complete with all the fullness of life and power that comes from God.

Now all glory to God, who is able, through his mighty power at work within us, to accomplish infinitely more than we might ask or think. (Ephesians 3:14–20 NLT)

The love of God truly does surpass knowledge, yet knowing this love is a sacred privilege of followers of Christ. Depression may make you feel dead inside but remember the God who loves you raises the dead.

7

Watch and Pray

"D o you think there might be some sin problem in your life?" my husband asked me one day about eight months into my journey after being hospitalized.

Furiously I snapped back with "Of course not. I can't control whether or not I'm depressed or the thoughts that come in my mind."

Learning that I needed to redirect my thoughts or replace them with Scripture had been my focus, leaving the thought of actually saying I was sorry to God and asking forgiveness nowhere to be found in my mind. I wanted to believe my husband as my spiritual leader, but I lacked the same conviction he did, which was difficult. There was no reason for me not to trust him, but depression was clouding my mind.

When my mental health journey began, I believed that if Jesus was enough, then I didn't need medication, medical treatments of any kind, or therapy. I used to believe that if I simply had enough faith, then I would not struggle.

But yet, even with faith, I did struggle. This left me in a terribly confusing state of mind where I was paralyzed out of complete confusion and never sought help for the sinister thoughts and despair that penetrated my mind and body. Then I went through an all-out breakdown, a couple hospitalizations and countless discussions with doctors, which swayed me to believe that my depression was only an illness that was completely out of my hands. This belief became dangerous because it convinced me that no responsibility fell to me in fighting it.

I was confused and I was struggling, and in hindsight, I can see how mental illness opened the door for the enemy to torture me with confusion. But aside from all of this, I kept doing the next right thing, and I was committed to staying in God's Word all the while complying with my doctors and therapists.

And while I was doing the best I knew how to do when it came to surviving and taking my thoughts captive, the Lord faithfully opened my eyes through Scripture of a key lacking ingredient in my journey toward mental health: repentance.

I found myself in the book of Romans, which clearly states the beautiful gospel of Jesus Christ. Paul shows through his letter that "In their union with Christ, all believers enjoy victory over sin, the law as the way of righteousness, and divine forgiveness for their sins."[1] Paul finally provides through his words to the Roman believers, "clear, practical guidelines on how believers should conduct their new lives in Christ and called them to make such a commitment."[2]

As I read through the book of Romans, chapter 6, which bore the title "Dead to Sin, Alive to God" in my Bible, arrested my struggling mind. I devoured the book as if it were the first time, even though it wasn't. The Word was proving to be alive and active and I was enthralled by each word. Near the middle of Romans is when the Holy Spirit convicted my heart for the sin I was unknowingly dismissing and I couldn't help but remember my husband's question regarding sin in my life.

"Maybe he was right," I started contemplating with a softened, more teachable heart.

Paul writes at the beginning of chapter 6, "We know that our old sinful selves were crucified with Christ so that sin might lose its power in our lives. We are no longer slaves to sin" (Romans 6:6 NLT).

> The power of sin has been broken in those who believe for their old self (lit., "old man," meaning who they were in Adam) was crucified and put to death with Christ. They were born into the world as sinners, with the result that their bodies were ruled by sin. Body of sin refers to the rule of sin, but without excluding the involvement of the personal self that lives through the body. Sin's rule, however, was broken when Christians died with Christ, and therefore they are no longer enslaved to sin. Paul does not argue that Christians do not sin at all (a view called sinless perfection); instead the tyranny, domination, and rule of sin have been defeated for them. This means that the normal pattern of life for Christians should be progressive growth in sanctification, resulting in ever greater maturity and conformity to God's moral law in thought and action.[3]

While reading the study notes in my Bible and applying them to the Scripture, what came to mind was the very thing that I felt had dominated and defeated me—the suicidal thoughts and urges I never once dreamed I'd need to repent from.

The idea of victory was nearly comical to me. And so, because I didn't see victory as a possibility, and I didn't see my thoughts as sinful, I was essentially choosing to walk in the darkness of sin, which is not what I'm called to as God's daughter.

I kept reading in Romans:

> For one who has died has been set free from sin. Now if we have died with Christ, we believe that we will also live with him. We know that Christ, being raised from the dead, will never die again; death no longer has dominion over him. For the death he died he died to sin, once for all, but the life he lives he lives to God. So

you also must consider yourselves dead to sin and alive
to God in Christ Jesus. (Romans 6:7–11 ESV)

God's Word opened the eyes of my heart to see just how
far I had drifted from walking in my true identity as a free,
victorious, powerful child of God who was completely dead
to sin. I was seeing the bondage I was in, and I was realizing
that there was no reason for me to stay there. "What has been
established, namely, is that believers are in principle dead to
sin and alive to Christ, must become the abiding conviction of
their hearts and minds, the takeoff point for all their thinking,
planning, rejoicing, speaking, doing. They must constantly
bear in mind that they are no longer what they used to be.
Their lives from day to day must show that they have not
forgotten this."[4]

It was becoming startlingly clear that the enemy enjoyed
persuading me into living a life enslaved to dark thoughts
when in reality, maybe I possessed more power over them than
I ever realized. I was captivated by the book of Romans as if I
were learning for the first time of all that has been given to me
through the death and resurrection of Christ. My mind was
being made new and transformation was in motion, and so, I
kept reading.

Paul continued, "Let not sin therefore reign in your mortal
body, to make you obey its passions. Do not present your
members to sin as instruments for unrighteousness, but present
yourselves to God as those who have been brought from death to
life, and your members to God as instruments for righteousness.
For sin will have no dominion over you, since you are not under
law but under grace" (Romans 6:12–14 ESV).

"The tension surfaces here between what God has already
accomplished and the responsibility of his people to obey. They
are still tempted by desires to sin and must not let those desires
gain control. Each day they must give themselves afresh to God."[5]

Brokenness flooded my heart as conviction painted many scenes of my past in a different light. I was truly aghast at just how many years, decades even, I allowed myself to be enslaved to sin when I didn't have to. And not just sin as in missing the mark of what I'm called to as a Christian, but the sin nature that is still in me.

There was a new brokenness for those believers I once knew that actually completed suicide. As helpless as I felt in my attempt to join them in their final act, I did stop. This is obedience in the fork in the road, and this is possible even with the most overwhelmingly intense sadness shaping the thoughts and actions of your body. If I could stop, so can you.

In this section of Scripture,

> Paul appealed to Christians to become in practice what they already are in status. They have already died to sin and are justified. Sin, however, still remains in their lives. Negatively, believers are to stop letting sin rule in their mortal bodies (subject to weakness and physical death) so that they obey sin's evil desires. Also, they are to stop presenting any part of their bodies (hands, feet, mouth, eyes, ears) to sin to be used as weapons or instruments of unrighteousness. Positively, believers should decisively surrender themselves and all parts of their bodies to God as weapons of righteousness.[6]

God was showing me that mental illness is not a sin, but the way that mental illness can be used to entice me to sin was becoming obvious. My mind's bent toward despair influenced my thoughts, what I would daydream about, my Google searches, my actions, and my obsessions. And while my natural inclination was to indulge in all of those things, I was seeing afresh that I didn't have to. Therapy taught me to understand why I was having suicidal thoughts as well. I learned that my mind had suppressed so much trauma in an effort to not feel pain. When my coping skills, such as trying to be perfect on the outside failed, suicidal thoughts became the firefighter that would react suddenly and remind me I did have an option to escape the pain. For some people drugs or alcohol may be the firefighter of choice, but for me, it was always death. When I combined the skills and understanding from therapy with the truth of God's Word, I found myself equipped in the best way possible to make the choice to walk away from the dark moments of temptation and walk in my true identity. My mind—a mind with diagnosed mental illness—has learned to think soberly and rationally in a new way, and that shows the beauty of God's Word, the power of the Holy Spirit, and the good gifts that therapy and medication if appropriate can be.

> In light of Paul's exhortation for us to consider ourselves "dead to sin," Merriam-Webster's Collegiate Dictionary has some interesting definitions of "dead" describing it as
>
>> lacking power to move, feel, or respond, incapable of being stirred emotionally or intellectually, unresponsive, inanimate, no longer functioning, lacking power or effect, no longer have interest, relevance or significance, no longer active, completely out of touch with.
>
> Now substitute some of those definitions in Paul's phrase "_____ *to sin*" and meditate upon this simple but great truth. Again we may not feel like this is true in light of your ongoing struggle with sin, but it is true.[7]

As a child of God, I can say with complete confidence that you are dead to sin. Sin has no power over you. Will you still struggle? Yes. Must you live a life of defeat as sin's slave to carry out whatever darkness it dictates? Absolutely not.

As I kept reading in Romans, Paul posed a question that invited a response: "Do you not know that if you present yourselves to anyone as obedient slaves, you are slaves of the one whom you obey, either of sin, which leads to death, or of obedience, which leads to righteousness?" (Romans 6:16 ESV).

I love how my Bible's study notes explained this verse, "Moral decisions still matter for Christians. Giving in to sin results in people becoming obedient slaves to sin. This kind of activity eventually leads to death, not implying that genuine believers can actually lose their salvation but that sinning leads them in that direction, away from full enjoyment of life with Christ."[8]

I sat back in my chair as hope filled my heart. Was repenting from sin the secret to the abundant life Jesus spoke of when He said, "The thief comes only to steal and kill and destroy. I came that they may have life and have it abundantly" (John 10:10 ESV)? Was repentance and walking in the newness of life that Jesus gave me though His death and resurrection the secret to joy in my sorrow? While the more I read, the more I was seeing life through a new lens, I was not done learning yet. And so, I continued on in Romans for weeks to come.

Finally in Romans 8, I read:

> So now there is no condemnation for those who belong to Christ Jesus. And because you belong to him, the power of the life-giving Spirit has freed you from the power of sin that leads to death. The law of Moses was unable to save us because of the weakness of our sinful nature. So God did what the law could not do. He sent his own Son in a body like the bodies we sinners have. And in that body God declared an end to sin's control over us by giving his Son as a sacrifice for our sins. He did this so that the just requirement of the law would be fully satisfied for us, who no longer follow our sinful nature but instead follow the Spirit.
>
> Those who are dominated by the sinful nature think about sinful things, but those who are controlled by the Holy Spirit think about things that please the Spirit. So letting your sinful nature control your mind leads to death. But letting the Spirit control your mind

leads to life and peace. For the sinful nature is always hostile to God. It never did obey God's laws, and it never will. That's why those who are still under the control of their sinful nature can never please God.

But you are not controlled by your sinful nature. You are controlled by the Spirit if you have the Spirit of God living in you. (And remember that those who do not have the Spirit of Christ living in them do not belong to him at all.) And Christ lives within you, so even though your body will die because of sin, the Spirit gives you life because you have been made right with God. The Spirit of God, who raised Jesus from the dead, lives in you. And just as God raised Christ Jesus from the dead, he will give life to your mortal bodies by this same Spirit living within you. Therefore, dear brothers and sisters, you have no obligation to do what your sinful nature urges you to do. For if you live by its dictates, you will die. But if through the power of the Spirit you put to death the deeds of your sinful nature, you will live. (Romans 8:1–13 NLT)

With razor sharp clarity, my mind shifted in regard to the suicidal thoughts that took up residence in my mind for years and deceived me into thinking that there was no way or even reason to get rid of them.

As I read the words of Romans over the span of a few months, it was painful at times, as if the Lord was performing surgery on my heart. There was correction, rebuke, frustration, and regret for my past mistakes. But God is so faithful and such a loving Father that along with the correction came reminders that I belong to Him such as "And because you belong to him, the power of the life-giving Spirit has freed you from the power of sin that leads to death" (Romans 8:2 NLT).

The new understanding gained from Scripture of the tension between my flesh and my spirit was incredible, but I still felt very much like my mind was in a war. I still needed to learn how to put my newly gained knowledge into practice.

Paul describes this tension that is found in every Christian for the entire span of their days on this earth in Romans when he said,

> And I know that nothing good lives in me, that is, in my sinful nature. I want to do what is right, but I can't. I want to do what is good, but I don't. I don't want to do what is wrong, but I do it anyway. But if I do what I don't want to do, I am not really the one doing wrong; it is sin living in me that does it. I have discovered this principle of life—that when I want to do what is right, I inevitably do what is wrong. I love God's law with all my heart. But there is another power within me that is at war with my mind. This power makes me a slave to the sin that is still within me. (Romans 7:18–23 NLT)

Reading Paul's words confirmed to me that my struggle between my flesh and my spirit wasn't as unusual as I once thought. I wanted to do what was right. I wanted to take my thoughts captive and make them obey Christ. I wanted to get to a place where I wouldn't even struggle in my flesh, but I was seeing that there might always be this battle because I live in a fallen body with a sin nature.

We all do and we all have since the first sin took place in the Garden of Eden. My mind was filling quickly with all this great head knowledge, but weariness was keeping me from really knowing how to walk in the freedom I was reading was possible.

As all of this swirled inside my mind and I tried to make sense of it all, I sat with my mentor where together we opened my journal and looked at what God was teaching me. I was learning to embrace vulnerability as a way to learn and improve rather than stay stuck in my questions and confusion.

These lessons altered my life and while I believed the Scriptures that were challenging my behavior, one day a few months after initially starting to study Romans, I remember scooting up close to my mentor, allowing her to read my heart in writing. I remember feeling weary as we looked at my journal together and discussed the battle I see myself, a believer, in. I know I have been freed from sin, yet my flesh still stumbles into sin at times. It's confusing, humbling, and embarrassing.

I felt as though I should be stronger by now or simply know better. And that's when she put her hands in the air and quoted Romans 7:24 to me with beautiful zeal. I was taken aback by her passion and memorization of the Word. I listened intently as she preached the gospel to me, a believer. She said, "Wretched man that I am! Who will deliver me from this body of death? Thanks be to God through Jesus Christ out Lord!" (Romans 7:24–25 ESV). I would go onto learn that some scholars believe that Paul may have in mind here a form of execution the Romans would use.

> A living man or woman was tied to a rotting corpse, face to face, mouth to mouth, limb to limb, with an obsessive exactitude in which each part of the body corresponded with its matching putrefying counterpart. Shackled to their rotting double, the man or woman was left to decay. To avoid the starvation of the victim and to ensure the rotting bonds between the living and the dead were fully established, the Etruscan robbers continued to feed the victim appropriately. Only once the superficial difference between the corpse and the living body started to rot away through the agency of worms, which bridged the two bodies, establishing a differential continuity between them, did the Etruscans stop feeding the living. Once both the living and the dead had turned black through putrefaction, the Etruscans deemed it appropriate to unshackle the bodies.[9]

What a disturbing punishment, but brilliant way to help us understand sin. The dead body was attached to the person who was alive in such a way that they eventually became one, turning black and being completely fused together. The corpse would then poison everything about the person being punished and ultimately kill them. This is what sin is and does. Sin attaches to you, poisons you, and leads to your death.

I felt that my suicidal thoughts were simply part of who I was. Being so engrained in me, they certainly tricked me into believing that they were at the core of who I was. But again, therapy helped me see that the suicidal thoughts were a very unhealthy coping skill that kept me alive in a sense by promoting the possibility of relief from pain. I needed to dig deep into the trauma with a therapist in order for them to eventually subside, but I also needed to understand that suicide is a sin and we are to make no provision for that.

And what does Paul say? "Wretched man that I am! Who will deliver me from this body of death? Thanks be to God through Jesus Christ our Lord!" It's not medication and it's not a cutting-edge medical treatment. It's not a therapist or a best friend that you confide in. Those are all amazing tools that have helped save my life, but Scripture answers the question for us in saying "Thanks be to God through Jesus Christ out Lord!" It's Jesus and only Jesus who can free us from the bondage of sin and empower us to walk in freedom even while residing in a body that has a sin nature.

Medicine and therapy are good gifts we are free to access as believers, but Jesus is our hope. So when we feel wretched— suffering, afflicted, miserable; suffering from spiritual or emotional misery[1]0—we must remember exactly Who it is that saves us from this sin that clings close and thrives in the dark.

Putting It All into Practice

I was doing my best to put into practice all the lessons I was learning about how I really do have more control over my thoughts than I once understood, and how the tension I feel, caught between my flesh and my spirit, is the normal

Christian experience, but something was still missing. And God, who is faithful to complete in us all that He begins, took me straight to the verse that would give me the missing puzzle piece.

I ended up in the book of Matthew where Jesus and His inner circle disciples (Peter, John, and James) accompanied him to garden to pray.

> Then Jesus went with them to a place called Gethsemane, and he said to his disciples, "Sit here, while I go over there and pray." And taking with him Peter and the two sons of Zebedee, he began to be sorrowful and troubled. Then he said to them, "My soul is very sorrowful, even to death; remain here, and watch with me." And going a little farther he fell on his face and prayed, saying, "My Father, if it be possible, let this cup pass from me; nevertheless, not as I will, but as you will." And he came to the disciples and found them sleeping. And he said to Peter, "So, could you not watch with me one hour? Watch and pray that you may not enter into temptation. The spirit indeed is willing, but the flesh is weak." (Matthew 26:36–41 ESV)

Noticing that Jesus spoke about the difference between the spirit and the flesh was new for me. Suddenly there was practical encouragement from Scripture that showed me what was missing in my life—prayer. Jesus instructed the disciples to watch and pray so they would not enter into temptation. Was I watching and praying? Could those two actions protect me from giving into temptation? Honestly at this point, my prayer life wasn't much to be proud of. Having drifted to a place where I really didn't even know how to pray anymore, I went back to the place where Jesus teaches us how, the Lord's Prayer.

There are six petitions that Jesus gives in the Lord's Prayer, with the final one being, "and lead us not into temptation, but deliver us from evil" (Matthew 6:13 ESV). I adopted that prayer as my own and began to wake up and immediately pray, "Lord, help me not give into temptation, and deliver me from any evil that is targeting me." With each passing day, I found strength in that prayer and an increased wakefulness so that I could be on guard against the devil's schemes.

> This final (sixth) petition addresses the disciples' battle with sin and evil. Lead us not into temptation—the word translated "temptation" (Gk. *peirasmos*) can indicate either temptation or testing. The meaning here most likely carries the sense, "Allow us to be spared from difficult circumstances that would tempt us to sin."
>
> Although God never directly tempts believers (James 1:13), He does sometimes lead them into situations to "test" them. In fact, trials and hardships will inevitably come to believers' lives, and believers should "count it all joy" (James 1:2) when trials come, for they are strengthened by them (James 1:3–4). Nonetheless, believers should never pray to be brought into such situations but should pray to be delivered from them, for hardship and temptation make obedience more difficult and will sometimes result in sin. Believers should pray to be delivered from temptation and led in "paths of righteousness."[11]

But what does it really mean to "watch"? "Watchfulness or watching indicates that the Christian is alert or vigilant in order to defend himself against a spiritual foe. He is properly prepared for any surprise or sudden change in his circumstances, and above all, in order that his fellowship with God in prayer may be undistracted and efficacious."[12]

Being watchful means to see the temptation coming, and prayer gives you the strength and grace to stand firm. Jesus's instruction to His disciples to watch and pray as a way to withstand temptation gave me the practical actions needed to apply and live out the theology I learned from Paul in the book of Romans.

Another place in Scripture where we see the combination of watchfulness and prayer as a strategy against the enemy is in the book of Nehemiah.

> Beginning in 605 BC, the Jews were taken from Jerusalem, the temple was destroyed (586 BC), and its resources were plundered by Kind Nebuchadnezzar of Babylon. However, in 538 BC, when Kind Cyrus of Persia conquered Babylon, he allowed his subjects to resume worship of their own gods, probably for political reasons, thus enabling the Jews to return to worship of the one true God. . . . Although the temple had been complete in 516 BC, the walls around Jerusalem were in shambles, and for this reason Nehemiah led his group back to Jerusalem. Through reforms he enacted, Nehemiah led his group back to Jerusalem. Through reforms he enacted, Nehemiah was able not only to restore the city walls but also to help preserve and challenge the spiritual condition of the people.[13]

In Nehemiah 4, we see how the Jews continue to build in spite of the opposition they faced. Everything was going well, and the wall was coming together beautifully. The people were working wholeheartedly, but like things sometimes go, Sanballat and others decided to interfere. "When Sanballat heard that we were rebuilding the wall, he became furious. He mocked the Jews before his colleagues and the powerful men of Samaria and said, 'What are these pathetic Jews doing? Can they restore it by themselves? Will they offer sacrifices? Will they ever finish it? Can they bring these burnt stones back to life from the mounds of rubble?'" (Nehemiah 4:1–2 CSB). They did not want to see the Jews succeed, so they chose to attack them.

> When Sanballat, Tobiah, and the Arabs, Ammonites, and Ashdodites heard that the repair to the walls of Jerusalem was progressing and that the gaps were being closed, they became furious. They all plotted together

to come and fight against Jerusalem and throw it into confusion. So we prayed to our God and stationed a guard because of them day and night.

In Judah, it was said: The strength of the laborer fails, since there is so much rubble. We will never be able to rebuild the wall.

And our enemies said, "They won't realize it until we're among them and can kill them and stop the work." When the Jews who lived nearby arrived, they said to us time and again, "Everywhere you turn, they attack us." So I stationed people behind the lowest sections of the wall, at the vulnerable areas. I stationed them by families with their swords, spears, and bows. After I made an inspection, I stood up and said to the nobles, the officials, and the rest of the people, "Don't be afraid of them. Remember the great and awe-inspiring Lord, and fight for your countrymen, your sons and daughters, your wives and homes." (Nehemiah 4:7–14 CSB)

Just as the enemies of Nehemiah and the Jews wanted to throw them into confusion, you too have an enemy who wants to confuse you, scare you, and kill you. Capitalizing on the intrusive thoughts you have is a classic scheme of the enemy.

Like Nehemiah, we must realize that if we focus on the enemy, rather than the work the Lord has placed in front of us, we will be discouraged and defeated. Have you ever felt like you have an enemy that sneaks in unannounced and then strikes when you least expect? Have you ever felt like everywhere you turn, you are attacked? I have.

Intrusive thoughts may accompany many types of mental illness, but you also have an enemy who is always planning for your destruction. If he can get your eyes off of the fruitful work in your lives—work done for the Lord—then he can kill you and stop the work.

No, the enemy can never snatch you from your Father's hand, and yes, you are eternally secure as God's child, but if satan can't steal your soul, he will certainly try to steal your fruitfulness. He will stop at nothing to extinguish your light on this earth. So what do we do? How did Nehemiah respond to their situation?

> Nehemiah listened to the concerns of his people, and he posted guards to protect the people from harm. Then he reminded his people that the Lord was on their side. Because God had commissioned their task, Nehemiah and the people could focus their attention on God instead of the enemies around them and thereby overcome the threats. Christians in subsequent generations must realize, as Nehemiah did, that no one can persevere through troubling times when she takes her focus off God.[14]

We must keep our eyes locked on Christ no matter how dark our hearts or minds feel.

Don't let the enemy use your sorrow to his advantage as a way to sideline you from the good works the Lord has prepared for you, but rather allow the solid food of Word of God to so fully saturate your mind that the schemes of the devil become obvious and your ability to distinguish between what is right and wrong becomes possible. "For someone who lives on milk is still an infant and doesn't know how to do what is right. Solid food is for those who are mature, who through training have the skill to recognize the difference between right and wrong" (Hebrews 5:13–14 NLT).

Nehemiah 4:15–20 (CSB) says,

> When our enemies heard that we knew their scheme and that God had frustrated it, every one of us returned to his own work on the wall. From that day on, half of my men did the work while the other half held spears, shields, bows, and armor. The officers supported all the people of Judah, who were rebuilding the wall. The laborers who carried the loads worked with one hand

and held a weapon with the other. Each of the builders had his sword strapped around his waist while he was building, and the one who sounded the ram's horn was beside me. Then I said to the nobles, the officials, and the rest of the people, "The work is enormous and spread out, and we are separated far from one another along the wall. Wherever you hear the sound of the ram's horn, rally to us there. Our God will fight for us!"

Everyone labored on the work before them with one hand yet held their weapon with the other. We see in the text that even though Nehemiah and the people asked and trusted God for protections, they also had their weapons nearby, ready to use to defend themselves from an enemy attack. God often accompanies his purposes through ordinary human means, and with mental illness in mind, we are to certainly pray and exercise faith in God, but it's also wise and good to take advantage of the ordinary means in which God has provided for you (for example, medication, nutrition, exercise, or therapy).

There comes a point where you, too, can recognize the enemy's scheme in your life with the sound mind that is yours, in spite of mental illness, through Christ Jesus. Through therapy, coping skills can help you change destructive habits in your thinking and through Scripture, wisdom and life can be found. It's not easy to persevere in the calling on your life when you battle mental illness and are opposed by an enemy that wants your witness stopped.

"Undoubtedly, these workers experienced fatigue, frustration, and fear; yet they stayed the course and attended to the work to which God had called them. Their witness is an encouragement for all the people of God, as Paul says, not to grow weary in doing good (Galatians 6:9). Perseverance, along with discernment to know when to persevere, are key attributes for the believer."[15]

So how did the workers complete their task? They watched and they prayed. They asked God for help, trusted in Him, and still wisely acted and utilized all that God provided for them. Charles Spurgeon describes this text as so: "In the text, I see two guards, first, prayer, 'We made our prayer unto God.' The second guard is watchfulness, 'We set a watch.' When I have spoken on these two subjects, I shall take, as my third topic, the two guards together. 'We prayed, and we set a watch.' We must have them both if we would defeat the enemy."[16]

We are people with both a flesh and a spirit. We are also people with both an enemy and a God who is sovereign over all. There will be tension in your life as a child of God, but that feeling of temptation to walk in the sinful nature of the flesh will not have dominion over you when you are watching and praying. The enemy cannot surprise attack you with the onslaught of despair and the urges to carry out suicide when you are awake and sober in your spirit. When therapy uncovers faulty thinking patterns in your mind, clarity leads to confidence which helps minimize the enemy's power over you. I'm praying over you in this journey, that you would "continue steadfastly in prayer, being watching in it with thanksgiving" (Colossians 4:2 ESV), and that as you continue persevering and walking in all that God has you doing, that you'd keep your eyes open, and every weapon of righteousness in your hand.

8

Clean Hands and a Pure Heart

Many of the years prior to pursuing mental health, I sat in church listening to beautiful sermons on the Lord, yet my thoughts were a million miles away. While honoring the Lord with my actions, I was simultaneously denying Him with my thoughts. I was a master at multitasking, or rather smiling on the outside, while secretly carrying out the act of killing myself in my mind. This came from a place a despair and is not unusual in those who live with depression.

I would play the scene over and over in my mind's eye, watching the death take place. I've died a thousand deaths in my mind without anyone knowing. I thought this was acceptable because I wasn't actually carrying out the act, but rather just secretly thinking about it in the hidden places no one could see.

But God gave my blind eyes sight to see the painful truth that His loving correction has given me the humility to swallow. He showed me the sinfulness and idolatry in the suicidal thinking buried deep inside my mind where I entertained them as if no one could see them. God, however, is always faithful to reveal truth to us and He brought me to a place of understanding that He "sees not as man sees; man looks on the outward appearance, but the Lord looks on the heart" (1 Samuel 16:7 ESV).

Every thought you think and every action you engage in is known by your Creator. "Even Death and Destruction hold no secrets from the LORD. How much more does he know the human heart!" (Proverbs 15:11 NLT).

Every death I died mentally, God intimately saw. Every imaginary suicide I've completed, the Lord has witnessed. I figured I was actually doing well because the imaginary suicides did not really steal my life, but deception skewed my thinking.

We can never forget that our enemy will take every inclination of our mind and bend it further toward darkness, for "He was a murderer from the beginning, and does not stand in the truth, because there is no truth in him. When he lies, he speaks out of his own character, for he is a liar and the father of lies" (John 8:44 ESV).

My secret fantasies of death were killing my faith without me even fully understanding. And yet, the Lord never gave up on me. He meets us where we are, but loves us too much to leave us there. If you are feeling like a lost cause, the Lord did not give up on me, and He has not given up on you either.

In my journey to mental health—not mental perfection, but mental stability—I have faithfully attended the women's Bible study at my church even when my heart was not in it. In fact, depression has often made staying in bed more appealing than going to church, however, one day at a time, as I made the decision to show up, the Lord faithfully and continually captured my attention with the mind-transforming Scripture that was being taught by the teacher.

In the year following my breakdown in Turkey, this women's Bible study was learning about the sermon Jesus gave located in Matthew 5–7. Tucked away in this great Sermon on the Mount is teaching regarding lust and adultery. At first glance, I pridefully thought, "This doesn't apply to me since I've never committed adultery."

As I paid attention to the lesson, however, God would sucker punch me with shocking conviction. You must remember, though, that while He is a God who convicts, He is also a God who comforts. He revealed glaring sin in my life, but the sufficient grace He supplied gave me the desire to not only turn from my ways, but the power to do so.

Starting in Matthew 5:27, Jesus said,

> You have heard that it was said, "You shall not commit adultery." But I say to you that everyone who looks at a woman with lustful intent has already committed adultery with her in his heart. If your right eye causes you to sin, tear it out and throw it away. For it is better that you lose one of your members than that your whole body be thrown into hell. And if your right hand causes you to sin, cut it off and throw it away. For it is better that you lose one of your members than that your whole body go to hell (Matthew 5:27–30 ESV).

While reading the Scripture and considering the original meaning of it, an unexpected application was made in my mind. If I'm looking at death with lustful intent, has my heart already committed it?

To lust after something is to yearn for it, or to direct your affections toward it. If I have yearned for death, I've lusted after it. According to Jesus, our hearts matter. Longing for my life to be over and going a step further and mentally going through with the act, was essentially the same as already having taken life. Yes, actually dying not only kills you, but kills your ministry and fruitfulness on this planet, but Jesus is after our hearts and wants to give us inside-out transformation that understands the severity of savoring suicidal thoughts and dying imaginary deaths, which very well could lead to actually going through with the act.

It's about your belief rather than your behavior. And Christlike behavior overflows from a heart that has been transformed through Jesus and brought to repentance through God's kindness.

Starting in James 4:4, we see more about adultery, but this time, it is spiritual in nature. James said,

> You adulterers! Don't you realize that friendship with the world makes you an enemy of God? I say it again: If you want to be a friend of the world, you make yourself an enemy of God. Do you think the Scriptures have no meaning? They say that God is passionate that the spirit he has placed within us should be faithful to him. And he gives grace generously. As the Scriptures say,
>
> "God opposes the proud,
>   but gives grace to the humble."
>
> So humble yourselves before God. Resist the devil, and he will flee from you. Come close to God, and God will come close to you. Wash your hands, you sinners; purify your hearts, for your loyalty is divided between God and the world. (James 4:4–8 NLT)

According to the Sermon on the Mount, this Scripture in James, and Scripture as a whole, we are called to more than physical purity, we are called to inner purity. God wants your heart, not just your good behavior.

Our mental faithfulness matters just as our physical faithfulness does, therefore we must do everything necessary to guard ourselves from engaging mentally in sinful acts of disobedience. If looking online for information on how to hurt yourself causes you to sin, "tear it out, and throw it away" so to speak by agreeing to restrictions being placed on your phone or computer for accountability about what you are searching for and longing after. If reading news stories of those who have followed through with suicide entice you to follow suit, "cut it off" as Jesus said in Matthew. Don't indulge in those stories that would conjure up the desire to be a copycat within you.

If having the means to carry out your death around the house makes it physically possible to complete what you've already committed mentally, then have a loved one lock everything dangerous up. Be radical in your pursuit of mental health and purity.

We must make no provision for sin. Savoring suicidal thoughts is lusting after the lie that the enemy has whispered to you and divides your loyalty between God and the world. Yes, medicine can decrease suicidal thoughts, and therapy is so important in getting to the root of why you are entertaining thoughts of self-harm, but nothing can deliver you or give you the ability to fight back like Jesus and the Word.

Living a divided life that seeks Jesus, but satisfies the longing for death by secretly contemplating it, is unstable, miserable, dangerous, and not walking in the light. Giving into suicidal rumination is committing spiritual adultery, for rumination lends itself to worshiping that which is thought about repeatedly.

Worshiping suicide in your mind while worshiping God with your lips is not God's plan for you. Mentally harping on your plans for death severs your devotion to God, life, hope, and joy. Just like physical adultery may start with an unfulfilled desire followed by a glance at that which is forbidden, so does spiritual adultery.

When we place our attention on anything other than God, and when we believe that anything can offer us more than God can, we are bowing down to an idol. We are committing adultery.

You are so very wanted and loved. So loved in fact, that the Lord wants you to walk in single-minded devotion to Him. Nothing you are thinking is hidden from Him,

For the LORD sees clearly what a man does,
  examining every path he takes.
An evil man is held captive by his own sins;
  they are ropes that catch and hold him.
He will die for lack of self-control;
  he will be lost because of his great foolishness.
                              (Proverbs 5:21–23 NLT)

But you, victorious one who has been given everything you need for life and godliness, you can walk in triumph. You belong to the Lord and you have been bought with a price. "For none of us lives to himself, and none of us dies to himself. For if we live, we live to the Lord, and if we die, we die to the Lord. So then, whether we live or whether we die, we are the Lord's" (Romans 14:7–8 ESV).

Perhaps you're reading this and still contemplating whether or not you're caught up in habitual, sinful thoughts that do not honor Jesus. Let's look at 1 John together. (I have added the bold text to show my application of scripture.)

This is the message [of God's promised revelation] which we have heard from Him and now announce to you, that God is Light [He is holy, His message is truthful, He is perfect in righteousness], and in Him there is no darkness at all [no sin, no wickedness, no imperfection]. If we say that we have fellowship with Him and yet walk in the darkness [of sin—**habitual suicidal ideation; contemplating suicide; fearing suicide**], we lie and do not practice the truth; but if we [really—**inside and out with no secret or hidden thoughts**] walk in the Light [that is, live each and every day in conformity with the precepts of God], as He Himself is in the Light, we have [true, unbroken] fellowship with one another [He with us, and we with Him], and the blood of Jesus His Son cleanses us from all sin [by erasing the stain of sin, keeping us cleansed from sin in all its forms and manifestations—**despair, anxiety, anger,**

fear, bitterness, and suicidal thoughts I dwell on]. If we say we have no sin [refusing to admit that we are sinners], we delude ourselves and the truth is not in us. [His word does not live in our hearts.] If we [freely] admit that we have sinned and confess our sins, He is faithful and just [true to His own nature and promises], and will forgive our sins and cleanse us continually from all unrighteousness [our wrongdoing, everything not in conformity with His will and purpose—**it is His will that my mind be transformed by the Word; that I take every thought captive; that I believe that I have the mind of Christ and not that I am fixated on death**]. If we say that we have not sinned [refusing to admit acts of sin—**believing I can't take suicidal thoughts captive and make them obedient to Christ; not acknowledging that sin can be our thoughts and not only our actions**], we make Him [out to be] a liar [by contradicting Him] and His word is not in us.

(1 John 1:5–10 AMP)

And this scripture as well:

We know [with confidence] that anyone born of God does not habitually sin (**this reminds me of a stronghold and my habitual suicidal thoughts**); but He (Jesus) who was born of God [carefully] keeps and protects him, and the evil one does not touch him. We know [for a fact] that we are of God, and the whole world [around us] lies in the power of the evil one [opposing God and His precepts]. And we [have seen and] know [by personal experience] that the Son of God has [actually] come [to this world], and has given us understanding and insight (**thank you, Lord!!**) so that we may [progressively **steadily moving forward** and personally] know Him who is true; and we are in Him who is true—in His Son Jesus Christ. This is the true God and eternal life. Little children (believers, dear ones), guard yourselves from idols (**my suicidal thoughts are an idol**) [false teachings, moral compromises, and anything that would take God's place in your heart]. (1 John 5:18–21 AMP)

A prayer I have prayed is: "God, forgive me for denying that my suicidal thoughts are sinful—not the initial thought, but the dwelling and savoring of the thought. The Truth is absolutely in me; please help me to live as if it were. Continue to show me where sin is a problem in my life, and help me to always have a deep brokenness for it." Perhaps this prayer resonates with you and can become your prayer as well. Like the Psalmist said, "May the words of my mouth and the meditation of my heart be acceptable to you, Lord, my rock and my Redeemer" (Psalm 19:14 CSB).

A mentally ill mind that mediates on that which is acceptable to the Lord is a beautiful way to show the world the transformative power of Scripture.

9

Abiding with Mental Illness

There were many days in my recovery, after my suicide attempt, that I felt nothing. Fatigue cast a shadow over everything that I did as emotional pain continued to pulse through my veins with a heartbeat like rhythm.

I had been reading the Bible sporadically in my pursuit of mental health, but I eventually developed a habit of waking up early, opening my Bible, and journeying through the pages from Genesis to Revelation in chronological order. It took one day of obedience which I then followed by another day. I was still very much bound like that woman in the synagogue, but also like her, I was doing the next right thing as I survived. For me, the next right thing was waking up every day and saturating my mind with Scripture, reminding myself that I could not be led by my emotions.

Medication certainly balanced the imbalance in my brain, therapy taught me healthy coping skills, and when I could muster up the motivation to exercise, my mind and mood benefitted greatly from embracing a healthy lifestyle. But nothing changed my life like spending consistent time with

God in His Word. The lessons I've shared within the covers of this book in your hands are the fruit of that discipline.

I didn't realize what was happening as days of doing the next right thing morphed into weeks and then months, but what was happening was the organic result of attaching myself to my Vine. I was abiding in Jesus. I was learning how to tarry, how to dwell as a daughter who was finding supernatural strength in her continued weakness by staying connected to her life source who is Christ.

Rather than surviving under the identity of broken, I was thriving as a beloved branch who was feasting on the nutrients found through faith in Christ. I was learning lessons and journaling them as a way to look back and remember all that God was teaching me. The process included pain due to unlearning lies and relearning truth, but each time a lie was cut out of my belief system, the fruit of faith grew stronger.

Life happens when you cease striving to survive mental illness in your own strength and thrust yourself into an existence of complete dependence on Jesus. Science offers so many wonderful gifts when it comes to improving the quality of life for those with mental illness, but Jesus is the only One who can bring life to the soul and a living hope where despair glosses over everything with darkness.

In John 15, we find the beloved Scripture about Jesus being the vine. While I didn't understand that I was finally abiding in Christ and therefore thriving in the midst of such brokenness of mind, this Scripture explains exactly what was happening as a result of staying connected to Jesus.

In the book of John, Jesus gives seven "I Am" statements with the final one being in John chapter 15. He says:

"I am the bread of life" (John 6:35, 41, 48, 51).
Jesus sustains us spiritually the way bread sustains us physically.

"I am the light of the world" (John 8:12). Jesus is the light that guides us in a world lost in darkness.

"I am the gate" (John 10:7, 9). Jesus is the Shepherd who protects his sheep from enemies.

"I am the resurrection and the life" (John 11:25). Death has no power over those who are in Christ.

"I am the good shepherd" (John 10:11, 14). Jesus watches over those who belong to Him.

"I am the way and the truth and the life" (John 14:6). All truth, knowledge, and direction, and life comes from Jesus.

"I am the true vine" (John 15:1, 5). The life of Christ flows in and through us when we attach ourselves to Jesus. Through this union, we bear fruit and glorify God.

John 15, found in the middle of beautiful goodbye known as the Farewell Discourse given by the Savior, is an illustration that not only teaches the importance of staying connected to Jesus, but the miraculous benefit from the union. "Jesus' allegory of the vine and the branches is at the very heart of the Farewell Discourse. The OT (Old Testament) frequently uses the vineyard or vine as a symbol for Israel, God's covenant people, especially in two 'vineyard songs' in Isaiah (Isa. 5:1–7; 27:2–6). However, Israel's failure to produce fruit resulted in divine judgement. Jesus, by contrast, is 'the true vine,' and his followers abide in him and produce fruit."[1] The section begins with Jesus speaking plainly to His disciples. He says: "I am the true vine, and my Father is the vinedresser. Every branch in me that does not bear fruit he takes away, and every branch that does bear fruit he prunes, that it may bear more fruit" (John 15:1–2 ESV). "The cultivation of vineyards was important to the life and economy of Israel. A golden vine adorned Herod's temple. When our Lord used this image, He was not introducing something new; it was familiar to every Jew."[2]

Jesus is clear in the two options He initially presents to His disciples by essentially saying "You can abide in me and bear fruit, or you can choose not to abide and not bear fruit." There really is no middle ground. And with mental illness, there really is no middle ground either. Perhaps you cannot choose whether or not you struggle with something like depression, but you can certainly choose whether or not you will submit and attach to Jesus or the enemy in your trial.

When you abide in Christ, you bear fruit. But what is this fruit? Let's look at Galatians for an example of the fruit that is produced from a life that has been not only been changed by the Holy Spirit, but also empowered by the Spirit. "But the fruit of the Spirit is love, joy, peace, patience, kindness, goodness, faithfulness, gentleness, and self-control. The law is not against such things" (5:22–23 CSB).

If we can't bear fruit apart from being connected to Him, then we can't expect to have true, lasting, supernatural joy in the midst of the sorrow, peace in the midst of anxiety, patience as you endure the ongoing depression, kindness when mental illness produces irritability, goodness when mental illness turns your gaze inward at the pain, faith when despair makes the future look bleak, gentleness when you feel inclined toward anger that God has allowed your suffering, and self-control when suicidal ideation, or the temptation to harm yourself in any way, rages in your mind.

> Fruitfulness is the result of the Son's life being reproduced in a disciple. The disciple's part is to remain. The word "remain," a key word in John's theology, is menō, which occurs 11 times in this chapter, 40 times in the entire Gospel, and 27 times in John's epistles. What does it

mean to remain? It can mean, first, to accept Jesus as Savior (cf. 6:54, 56). Second, it can mean to continue or persevere in believing (8:31 ["hold" is remain]; 1 John 2:19, 24). Third, it can also mean believing, loving obedience (John 15:9–10). Without faith, no life of God will come to anyone. Without the life of God, no real fruit can be produced: Neither can you bear fruit unless you remain in Me.[3]

But if you're remaining in Jesus, why does God, the vinedresser, need to prune you? Because there is always more fruitfulness possible. To prune means to purify or cleanse from filth with the purpose of even more fruit being produced. Pruning, however, is painful.

> The vinedresser prunes the branches in two ways: he cuts away dead wood that can breed disease and insects, and he cuts away living tissue so that the life of the vine will not be so dissipated that the quality of the crop will be jeopardized. In fact, the vinedresser will even cut away whole bunches of grapes so that the rest of the crop will be of higher quality. God wants both quantity and quality.[4]

Before my breakdown and hospitalization in Turkey, I thought I was fruitful. I was to an extent. I was doing great things for God and seeing the fruit of the Spirit flow from my life, but eventually my ability to keep pressing on in my own strength, and completely ignoring the trauma and illness in my mind and body, dissipated. When I was removed from the obvious ministry in my life and found myself in and out of hospitals, as well as at home trying to simply survive, my perspective of what ministry needed to look like was being pruned.

Both hospitalizations brought a deeper level of humility, resulting in a more genuine Christlikeness in me. Each morning I woke up and chose to start my day with God in His Word and in prayer, I was learning the beauty found in relationship with my Father and that through the power of the Spirit, the self-control necessary to do that which I did not want to do, was possible. When I choose to believe that there really is no condemnation in Christ, then I am saying no to shame and being pruned to live a more free and fruitful existence.

Pruning hurts, but it comes from God's heart of love for you, and the alternative is rejecting redemption in Christ and therefore being thrown away and burned. Because you, Child of God (regardless of whether or not you live with a mental illness) were created to be fruitful, pruning is God's loving plan for perfecting you. And when God is your delight bearing fruit in every season, even a season of depression, becomes possible, for

> Blessed is the one
> who does not walk in step with the wicked
> or stand in the way that sinners take
> or sit in the company of mockers,
> but whose delight is in the law of the LORD,
> and who meditates on his law day and night.
> That person is like a tree planted by streams of water,
> which yields its fruit in season
> and whose leaf does not wither—
> whatever they do prospers.
>
> (Psalm 1:1–3)

While Jesus was talking to His disciples, He continued: "Already you are clean because of the word that I have spoken to you. Abide in me, and I in you. As the branch cannot bear fruit by itself, unless it abides in the vine, neither can you, unless you abide in me" (John 15:3–4 ESV). Abiding is simply a continual personal relationship with Jesus, and that union will be characterized by trust, prayer, obedience, and joy. Without this union, you cannot bear fruit.

Practically speaking, when you wake up for the day and the lies immediately attempt to lure you away, yet you focus your mind on God by lamenting all that is discouraging you, you are abiding in Christ. You are choosing to trust that the God of your salvation hears your cries and will act on your behalf. When you obey God and take your toxic thoughts captive and make them obedient to Christ, despite the deeply dark emotions you feel, you are abiding in Christ. When you find your joy in the strength of the Lord while suffering intense sadness, you are abiding in Christ.

When depression demands so much of you that you find yourself fatigued in bed, your faith and trust in Jesus, as you endure, is bearing fruit. When dark thoughts inspire imaginings that would offer relief from your fallen body, and you cry out to God for help setting your mind on things above, you are bearing fruit.

When anxiety causes you to panic and you find yourself on your knees in prayer, confessing your fears and asking for more faith, you are bearing fruit. When in your brokenness, you tell someone how God's grace is sustaining you and how Jesus is your hope, you are bearing fruit. And when the Holy Spirit reveals sin in your life, and you cooperate by turning away from that sin to follow the ways of Jesus, you are bearing fruit. Truly, the secret to hope in despair, joy in sorrow, and obedience in brain fog is dwelling with Jesus—staying connected to Him.

I'm not here to tell you I have always done this perfectly or that it is an easy task for me, but I am here to genuinely express to you that abiding in Jesus has been the way I have not only survived but thrived. Bearing fruit beautifully bears witness to your union with Him. Even believers with broken minds can bear much fruit when they stay intimately connected to the vine, so if you are reading this and the thought of pursing a relationship with anyone, including Jesus, is so very daunting, please know that while I understand, I can always testify that it is worth it.

It's hard, but not impossible to abide in Christ while simultaneously living with sorrow, grief, or mental illness. Let's find our home in Him, remembering that He is the source of all life within the broken minds that naturally gravitate toward the grave. The enemy may bend your mind toward death, but you do not have to yield.

His Words in You

In the months following the hospitalizations where I was learning and growing and sometimes failing, I remember one night where I was presented the opportunity to practice all I had been learning. I woke up in a panic as I squinted my eyes to see in the darkness around 3:00 a.m. "Greater is he who is in me than he who is in the world" was my desperate whisper as I clutched the sides of my broken brain. "Help me, God," I thought in my moment of need. I was in bed while my family slept soundly, yet my mind was anything but sound.

I was cooperating with a psychiatrist and talking to a therapist, but even after utilizing those good gifts, darkness continued to linger.

Irrational thinking in that moment of sleepiness seemed rational in my mind. Death's allure attracted me like a moth to the light. "And no wonder, for Satan himself masquerades as an angel of light" (2 Corinthians 11:14). I was in a sudden battle to live, but in that moment of panic at the intersection of life and death, the Spirit brought to mind a verse I knew.

"The one who is in you is greater than the one who is in the world" (1 John 4:4).

I held onto that verse as if my life depended on it, which really it did. With eyes clamped closed and my hands clutching the sides of my head, I whispered the truth from that verse on repeat. With each repetition, that seed of truth grew, eventually breaking through the hard ground and reaching for the light. Fruit was being produced in my moment of panic as my faith was being exercised and the words hidden in my heart were my weapon in the battle.

As I proclaimed the greatness of the Spirit in me compared to the enemy in this world, panic subsided. I still felt the sadness, but the fear of myself was gone and by depending on God, I won the victory over another moment.

Moments become days which then in turn become months and then years and before long, thriving in spite of depression has become possible. The idea of God's words abiding in us is no new idea. Jesus said to his disciples: "If you remain in me and my words remain in you, ask whatever you wish, and it will be done for you" (John 15:7). We remain in Him, but don't miss that His words must also remain in us. It does not mean to just memorize Scripture, for even satan can do that. Scripture must be fed to the mind so it can take root in our hearts and as a result, influence the way we think, act, believe, and speak. And in order for that to happen, we must be students of the Word.

Your heart cannot cling to and savor what your mind does not know. His words abiding in you looks like reading Truth, taking it in, dwelling on it, and asking God to transform you from the inside out. When the words of God abide in you, they become this safeguard against temptation and a sword to demolish lies, for we are even told to take up "the sword of the Spirit, which is the word of God" (Ephesians 6:17).

Your mental illness may seem like your enemy, but never forget of the greater enemy that lurks in the shadows. You must remember to "Put on the whole armor of God, that you may be able to stand against the schemes of the devil. For we do not wrestle against flesh and blood, but against the rulers, against the authorities, against the cosmic powers over this present darkness, against the spiritual forces of evil in the heavenly places" (Ephesians 6:11–12 ESV). There is no greater example of living this out practically than our Savior Himself. As Jesus was being tempted in the wilderness,

The tempter came and said to him, "If you are the Son of God, command these stones to become loaves of bread." But he answered, "It is written,

" 'Man shall not live by bread alone,
but by every word that comes from the mouth
of God.'" (Matthew 4:3–4 ESV)

In a moment of desperation, Jesus could have spoken new revelations or said nothing, but He chose the cling to the written Word as His sword in the battle. We cannot live on bread—natural means—alone. We cannot rely solely on medication or any other means that has been provided for us in the wilderness, but only by the Word of God. Jesus knew this and He lived this. So for us, what does that look like? It means getting up and opening up the Bible and reading even when we don't feel like it or even when only a few words is the best we can do, because the Word really does transform our thinking and become our weapon in war.

If we look back to John 5, we can see the mounting Jewish opposition toward Jesus. In John 5:37–40 (CSB), Jesus said, "The Father who sent me has himself testified about me. You have not heard his voice at any time, and you haven't seen his form. You don't have his word residing in you, because you don't believe the one he sent. You pore over the Scriptures because you think you have eternal life in them, and yet they testify about me. But you are not willing to come to me so that you may have life."

We see in these words spoken by Christ, that the study of Scripture does not in and of itself save you. The Bible, rather, attests to the One who does give life and salvation, Jesus. Because it's through studying the Word of God that we come to learn about and understand Jesus, the study of the Bible should result in genuine belief in Jesus followed by obedient action. Merely acquiring biblical knowledge does not save you or in our case help you endure life that is marred by mental illness. Genuine faith, which grows from a transformed life and relationship with Jesus Himself, is what saves you and gives you all the power you need to persevere even in the most painful of times.

So when we have Christ's words abiding in us, we believe. And belief is everything. If Scripture abides in you, you will believe the Scripture and more importantly, the One who spoke it. When the Word of God abides in you, you believe in Jesus and attach yourself to Him. The fiery flames of depression cannot extinguish a faith that is anchored securely in Christ, directing the eyes to focus on the eternal rather than the current suffering. Sometimes God delivers us from the trial, but sometimes He uses the trial to deliver us.

The king of Babylon commanded everyone to bow down and worship the golden statue he commanded to be built, and insisted three Jewish men be thrown in the furnace when they refused. These men bravely said, "Our God whom we serve is able to deliver us from the burning fiery furnace, and he will deliver us out of your hand, O king. But if not, be it known to you, O king, that we will not serve your gods or worship the golden image that you have set up" (Daniel 3:17–18 ESV).

In the face of death, these men held onto truth without even the promise of deliverance. They knew God could save them, but were never given the assurance that in His divine wisdom, He would.

At the king's command, they were bound and helpless. I still feel that way often, and I'm guessing you do too. Like the bound daughter of Abraham, who was unable to help herself, so they must have felt. They chose to trust God as they were literally thrown into a fiery furnace that was heated up seven times hotter than normal. But the most amazing thing happened, as they walked around in flames, a fourth heavenly being was seen with them.

When everyone "gathered together and saw that the fire had not had any power over the bodies of those men. The hair of their heads was not singed, their cloaks were not harmed, and no smell of fire had come upon them" (Daniel 3:17 ESV). In fact, the fire freed them from their bondage. Again, sometimes God delivers us from the trial, but sometimes He uses the experience of the trial to deliver us. When you are abiding in Christ, and receiving everything you need from Him, no depression will singe you, no anxiety will burn you, and there will be no smell of suicide on you, dear child of God. The self-dependence that once bound me has been burned off me in the fire. It has been hard and scary at times, but it has been a deliverance in my life that I continue to walk in.

The king exclaimed, "Praise to the God of Shadrach, Meshach, and Abednego! He sent his angel and rescued his servants who trusted in him" and even went on to declare, "For there is no other god who is able to deliver like this" (Daniel 3:28–29 CSB).

Mental illness puts a target on your back. With a mind bent toward despair, the enemy knows hopelessness is an easy temptation. Hopelessness threatens faith and can leave even a child of God searching for a way to escape the pain no matter the cost.

But here's the thing, even in the fiery furnace of depression, God is faithful to never forsake. When you fix your focus on Christ in your crisis, His faithfulness will empower you to fight the good fight of faith. Perhaps He doesn't rescue you from having to go through the experience of the flames, but He never leaves you during the fight. If our trust in Him is not dependent on our circumstances, others will undoubtedly glorify the Lord. Even the king of Babylon declared that there was no other god besides our God who can deliver like He does.

And when you do come out of the furnace of affliction, know that even if the illness aspect remains—for we do live in fallen bodies—the enemy's stronghold can be destroyed through Jesus. We can walk spiritually unharmed and without even a hint of the smell of fire on us.

Living with mental illness is exactly that, living with it. It doesn't just go away. On good and bad days alike, it's there. It's the backdrop for every decision, feeling, and thought. It's the lens the world is seen through. Some days things happen, people say things, or someone treats you a certain way that flips the switch to a full-on trauma response. Physical symptoms surge through your being, and suddenly you find yourself diving fast into a dark war zone where hope is bleak and the good fight of faith intensifies. Underneath your smile, a battle rages in secret places no one sees. Except God, because He is the God Who Sees.

How do we not lose hope? We feed our aching minds with the nourishment found in God's Word—even when pain makes opening up the Bible seem less than appetizing. We must abide in the Word, remain in it, tarry there. Jesus also said, "It is the Spirit who gives life; the flesh is no help at all. The words that I have spoken to you are spirit and life" (John 6:63 ESV).

The flesh, which includes the intellect, will, and emotions of humans, is completely unable to produce true spiritual life on its own. Only the Spirit, who works powerfully in and through the words of Christ, can accomplish this. The words of Jesus that are to abide in us, have the miraculous ability to awaken the unseen spiritual life deep within you that you long for.

Secret to Joy

As Jesus continued talking to His disciples about the importance of abiding in Him, He said,

> By this my Father is glorified, that you bear much fruit and so prove to be my disciples. As the Father has loved me, so have I loved you. Abide in my love. If you keep

my commandments, you will abide in my love, just as
I have kept my Father's commandments and abide in
his love. These things I have spoken to you, that my joy
may be in you, and that your joy may be full.

(John 15:8–11 ESV)

Jesus knew joy and He clung to it through horrors we can
only imagine. It is written in Hebrews 12:2 (CSB), "For the
joy that lay before him, he endured the cross, despising the
shame, and sat down at the right hand of the throne of God."
Jesus looked forward with joy to all that was coming which
empowered him to endure the gruesome, shameful, horrifying
cross. "For consider him who endured such hostility from
sinners against himself, so that you won't grow weary and give
up" (Hebrews 12:3 CSB).

God is glorified by our fruit-bearing endurance and in
turn, our discipleship is proven. God loves us and calls us to
abide in that love. But what kind of love allows such tragic
suffering? What type of love allows mental illness? A Father's
love. A love so deep that it will hold back from stopping pain
out of the divine knowledge that it is for your ultimate good
and His glory.

God intends that the miraculous, empowering joy that was
set before Christ and helped Him persevere, be your joy. To be
Christian is to fully embrace every aspect of Christ whether it
be the suffering, the resurrection, or the future coming. Jesus's
eyes looked forward with hope and expectation of all the joy that
was coming and that gave Him the strength to keep going even
though His heart's cry was "My Father! If it is possible, let this
cup of suffering be taken away from me" (Matthew 26:39 NLT).

If you are a born-again believer, then no matter how horrific
your suffering is today, the future that awaits you is perfect and
nothing but pure joy. This joyful sorrow belonged to Christ as
He suffered unthinkable pain, and this joy can belong to you
as well.

We must remember, though, that this joy is not something we can just muster up in our own strength, but rather a fruit of the Spirit that is produced through our union with Christ. There is just no true joy apart from relationship with Jesus. When God allows mental illness in your mind and calls you to take each suicidal thought captive while setting your mind on things above rather than things of this earth, and you obey, it is for your joy. When God has not stopped depression in your mind and body and prompts you to use this as a way to share about Jesus, and you humbly do so, it is for your joy, and not just a little joy, but that your joy may be full, that even in your sorrow, you may be joyful.

I know the pain in your life is real and can feel unbearable, but the joy that was before Jesus, or rather the hope of the resurrection He looked forward to, was the joy that kept Him resolved to endure the pain of the cross. And so it is with us.

My prayer for you is that you will not deny your pain, but that in it, you will experience the joy that comes from looking forward with hope to the day that Jesus makes all things new and right and mental illness ceases to exist. This day will come, and it will be glorious.

10

Unhindered Hope

When the hand of depression presses, the depth of pain feels unbearable. Depression locks the mind away in darkness, sometimes even blocking the ability to attach words to distress. There are times when a heavy sigh speaks a thousand words as it escapes the lungs. And God can interpret each breath, pregnant with emotion, exhaled from those who feel like the living dead.

God hears your cry for help, even when it comes in the form of a sigh. God listens when your prayers flow in the form of distraught groans and heavy breathing. He responds to your breathing toward Him in the valley of the shadow of death, even when confusion clouds your understanding of what you need. Your sighs are not meaningless movement of breath when directed at God, but rather hope-filled signs of life.

The Holy Spirit residing in you, child of God, "helps us in our weakness. For example, we don't know what God wants us to pray for. But the Holy Spirit prays for us with groanings that cannot be expressed in words" (Romans 8:26 NLT). Faith-filled, wordless groans of the humble are more powerful that exquisite prayers of the wordsmith who just wants to appear holy. If you are sighing, hold fast. Jesus has made a way, the Holy Spirit intercedes, and God listens.

Suffering and sighing must have been intimately known by the apostle Paul who wrote Romans 8:6. And your suffering is no accident. In fact, the God who told Moses "There is no god besides me. I put to death and I bring to life, I have wounded and I will heal, and no one can deliver out of my hand" (Deuteronomy 32:29) is the same God who knows the inner workings of your brain. The enemy can attack us, but any and all power He possesses has been allotted to him by God. Your mental illness has been allowed by God because His ways are higher than ours. Satan can absolutely torment, but every attempt he makes at taking down a child of God is simply turned into an instrument for strengthening our faith in God's providence. The Lord's primary goal for His people is not health, wealth, and ease. It's holiness, godliness, and a beautiful dependence which is often manifested when all is lost but hope, which no one can take from you.

Paul knew this living hope, but it came at a price. In a letter to the Corinthians, he wrote: "For we do not want you to be unaware, brothers, of the affliction we experienced in Asia. For we were so utterly burdened beyond our strength that we despaired of life itself. Indeed, we felt that we had received the sentence of death" (2 Corinthians 1:8–9 ESV). Paul transparently shared how the affliction was beyond their strength. They felt crushed and wholly without resource. It was overwhelming and exceeded their ability to endure. I've felt this in my own life, and I'm guessing you have too.

As I began hemorrhaging after the birth of my third child, I was certain I was dying. While a team rushed to save my life, my husband was prepared to lose me. As nurses and doctors swirled around me, I stared at the white ceiling convinced I was breathing my last breaths this side of heaven. When I gained consciousness, I was surprised I was alive, and traumatized.

Paul's experience is the definition of a traumatic event. The story doesn't end there in hopelessness but knowing a traumatized human penned much of the New Testament gives a different perspective when you see how Paul encouraged others toward faith, hope, and love. When life experiences are so difficult that we think they will kill us, Paul's life is one worth remembering and imitating. The trauma he survived not only makes him more relatable, but the resurrection power of Christ shines through him. Charles Spurgeon, known as the "Prince of Preachers" reminds me of Paul in the way he views suffering.

> I often feel very grateful to God that I have undergone fearful depression of spirits. I know the borders of despair, and the horrible brink of that gulf of darkness into which my feet have almost gone; but hundreds of times I have been able to give a helpful grip to brethren and sisters who have come into that same condition, which grip I could never have given if I had not known their deep despondency. So, I believe that the darkest and most dreadful experience of a child of God will help him to be a fisher of men if he will but follow Christ.[1]

While we cannot know for sure if Paul suffered from Post-traumatic Stress Disorder, I certainly think it is appropriate to contemplate how the intense hardships he endured were indeed traumatic. As Paul continued writing to the Corinthians, he described in detail the abuse he endured as a follower of Jesus.

> He was whipped thirty-nine times.
> He was beaten with rods.
> He received a stoning.
> He was shipwrecked three times.
> He spent a day and night in the open sea.
> He faced the danger of rivers.
> He faced danger from his own people, the Gentiles, the city, the wilderness, robbers, the sea, and false believers.
> He went without sleep.

He went hungry.
He was thirsty.
He was cold and went without clothing.

Paul's relationship with trauma must have been complicated. Becoming a follower of Jesus, after he actively persecuted Christians, would have attached a unique grief to his memories. Trauma is not always something done to you but can also stem from your own actions. Before his conversion, he spent his life imprisoning men and women in a violent attempt to demolish the church. When he was still actively working against God, it is said that he was "still breathing threats and murder against the disciples of the Lord. He went to the high priest and requested letters from him to the synagogues in Damascus, so that if he found any men or women who belonged to the Way, he might bring them as prisoners to Jerusalem" (Acts 9:1–2 CSB).

As a believer, he was a devoted man of God with a past that couldn't have been easily forgotten. Perhaps he was not a slave to debilitating flashbacks, but the graphic and disturbing memories in his human mind would have certainly been a target of satan's temptation toward shame, despair, and condemnation.

While reading Paul's account of the affliction they endured in Asia, I couldn't help but notice the frankness in which he wrote. My natural inclination has been to allow shame to lock away any story of trauma that has been written into my narrative. When we deny the pain we are dealing with, or the sickness that is ravaging our bodies, we rob God the glory due His name in the way He helps us.

The mentally ill child of God who endures unrelenting sadness shows all the sustaining grace of God. The anxious believer who asks others for prayer and then walks in the peace granted by God will only deepen the faith of those who prayed. The suicidal Christian who chooses to endure with a mind that is trying to kill them shows faith in God's plan over taking their life into their own hands.

We must not gloss over the darkness, assuming it will make a pretty story that will draw others to Jesus. No, the hurting world can't identify with the phony smiles of filtered lives and edited stories. There is beauty when the afflicted see the brokenness you have gone through, or continue to go through, and how the Lord sustains you.

Sometimes God delivers the hurting from their pain, but sometimes He doesn't. If we wait until the suffering stops to share our stories, assuming a tidy story equals a powerful story, we may live our entire lives and never once share our stories. Our suffering can coexist with a fruitful life that is sustained by God's grace, which testifies to the joyful sorrow of the Christian experience. Yes, Paul experienced trauma that was so scary and so hard that they despaired of life itself. But like all of our stories, there is purpose in our pain which allows joy to infuse the struggling believer with the strength of the Lord.

Paul tied the trauma to purpose by sharing,

> Indeed, we felt that we had received the sentence of death, so that we would not trust in ourselves but in God who raises the dead. He has delivered us from such a terrible death, and he will deliver us. We have put our hope in him that he will deliver us again while you join in helping us by your prayers. Then many will give thanks on our behalf for the gift that came to us through the prayers of many. (2 Corinthians 1:9–11 CSB)

He made it known that his trust was in the God who raises the dead. He understood that the depth of their suffering showed them they could not trust themselves. He acknowledged the way God has delivered them in the past, which gave them eyes of hope for future deliverance. That hope begets endurance, which is so necessary in the Christian life. Paul also reveals the power of prayer and how the affliction, along with their hope in the Lord, surrounded by prayers of others, results in the thanksgiving of many. Ultimately, the result in God being glorified.

What would happen if we started to embrace suffering and walk through it in community? We would see the power of shame broken; prayer lives strengthened; and voices of thanksgiving rise in one accord to the God of all hope. Paul accepted suffering as a natural part of his life as a follower of Christ. He not only accepted it, but his heavenly perspective gave him eyes to see how everything that happened to him was for his good, and the good of others. But let's not forget his humanity. Throughout Scripture, his trials were not minimized, but rather recorded as an eternal testimony.

We don't have to gloss over or minimize our pain either. The miracle is seen when others know of your weakness and watch God empower you to do all things through Christ who gives you strength. There is purpose in your pain. It feels like it will last forever, but through Jesus, it will end one day. "Therefore we do not give up. Even though our outer person is being destroyed, our inner person is being renewed day by day. For our momentary light affliction is producing for us an absolutely incomparable eternal weight of glory. So we do not focus on what is seen, but on what is unseen. For what is seen is temporary, but what is unseen is eternal" (2 Corinthians 4:16–18 CSB).

Near the end of Acts, we find Paul arrested by Jews, under the approval of the Sanhedrin, plotting to kill him. Eventually, Paul, as a Roman citizen, appealed to Caesar, resulting in a long and treacherous journey, by ship, toward Rome. As the voyage grew increasingly more dangerous, Paul declared,

> "Men, I can see that this voyage is headed toward disaster and heavy loss, not only of the cargo and the ship but also of our lives." But the centurion paid attention to the captain and the owner of the ship rather than to what Paul said. Since the harbor was unsuitable to winter

in, the majority decided to set sail from there, hoping somehow to reach Phoenix, a harbor on Crete facing the southwest and northwest, and to winter there.

(Acts 27:10–12 CSB)

Can you imagine the terror of knowing you were headed toward disaster, and possibly death, and no one would listen?

Because of past trauma, hypervigilance has been woven into the way I function, which lends to my imagination wondering if Paul was hypervigilant as well. Was he terrified? Was he on edge? While God worked amazing miracles in and through Paul, he was in fact, completely human. His body and mind would have been just as prone to react to trauma like any other human. We cannot read his writings and place him on a pedestal as someone whose intimate relationship with God would have protected his brain from what science tells us today happens after trauma.

"Trauma results in a fundamental reorganization of the way mind and brain manage perceptions. It changes not only how we think, but also our very capacity to think."[2] What was going on in Paul's mind, body, and brain as he saw impending doom, and no one listened? What a helpless feeling that must have been.

Eventually, because of being so violently storm-tossed, they threw cargo overboard. Acts 27:20 gives us a glimpse into the despair those on the ship succumbed to. "When neither sun nor stars appeared for many days and the storm continued raging, we finally gave up all hope of being saved."

All hope was abandoned.

Mental illness can certainly leave one feeling violently storm-tossed. Like a roaring tempest, a deep bout with depression or a panic attack can come on suddenly, leaving you feeling bruised and battered. The darkness becomes so black that any glimpse of blue sky—of hope—is blotted out.

Feelings of being unprepared, overwhelmed, isolated, confused, and terrified are not uncommon when the storms of life rage. Uncontrollable, overflowing tears mimic heavy, unrelenting rain. Like a trauma-infused flashback, a storm can appear out of nowhere, lifting just as quickly as it arrived. But a lifted storm does not equate to a peaceful mind, body, and brain. "Traumatized people keep secreting large amounts of stress hormones long after the actual danger has passed."[3]

Everything on the outside might appear normal, but the inner life of the traumatized person, believer or not, might still be in the middle of a storm. Storms can bring with them floods that can wipe out relationships, once held beliefs, faith, and even life itself. The darkness can be so oppressive that it's as though both sun and stars are completely hidden for days, weeks, and months on end. When the no small tempest of mental illness lays upon you, it's easy to abandon all hope of being saved.

This is the hopelessness the passengers on the ship headed to Rome found themselves entertaining, and this is where I have found myself in my own struggle with depression, anxiety, and PTSD. Untreated, undiagnosed mental illness can be lived with, but sooner or later, the stress catches up to you and one can easily run out of coping skills. The pain becomes so overwhelming that death can become the escape of choice and satan always celebrates abandonment of all hope.

Loss of all hope is not where this story ends, however, and it's not where your story ends either.

> Since they had been without food for a long time, Paul then stood up among them and said, "You men should have followed my advice not to sail from Crete and sustain this damage and loss. Now I urge you to take courage, because there will be no loss of any of your lives, but only of the ship. For last night an angel of the God I belong to and serve stood by me and said,

'Don't be afraid, Paul. It is necessary for you to appear before Caesar. And indeed, God has graciously given you all those who are sailing with you.' So take courage, men, because I believe God that it will be just the way it was told to me. But we have to run aground on some island." (Acts 27:21–26 CSB)

Paul, the man of God who has been through unthinkable horror in his life, was able to stand up among the storm-battered men and urge them to take courage. The storm was no less severe for Paul, and yet his reaction in the midst of the trial is opposite of the other passengers. But how could he do this? How could he, in such a physically and emotionally demanding trial, have the sober mind to call men to courage? The secret is found in his powerful words: "The God I belong to and serve stood by me" (Acts 27:23 CSB).

When you know who you belong to and who stands next to you, miraculous strength manifests itself in our mortal bodies. Our actions originate in our minds. There was tremendous power in the faith Paul possessed. A believer so convinced in their mind of their blood-bought identity as a child of God, will not crumble under the sorrows of life, the difficulty of living with mental illness, and grief that is inexpressible with words. Not only will they survive, but they will be a catalyst in those around them in choosing faith over fear. Paul never let go of the goodness of God, saying "What's more, God in his goodness has granted safety to everyone sailing with you" (Acts 27:24 NLT). When the storms of mental illness are raging, we must follow Paul's example:

- Paul remembered who he belonged to.
- Despite everything, he called God good.
- He believed God would keep His promises.

Out of the discipline of doing these three things, despite what his heart may have felt, came hope and encouragement to those around him. He was a living example of these words of Peter: "Therefore, with your minds ready for action, be sober-minded and set your hope completely on the grace to be brought to you at the revelation of Jesus Christ" (1 Peter 1:13 CSB).

Although they would survive, like Paul said, they had "run aground on some island" (Acts 27:26). God revealed to Paul that they would live, but in God's wisdom and will, there would still be a shipwreck.

I think back to when I lived in Turkey and served the Lord. I knew something was wrong in my mind, but I felt helpless and hopeless that help would ever come. I just kept my hand to the plow and tried my best to encourage others from a place of extreme emptiness and discouragement.

Why would God go to such extremes as to allow me to hit rock bottom and end up in a Turkish psychiatric hospital without access to the Bible or contact with the outside world? The experience carried with it its own form of trauma. But what if I hadn't experienced that shipwreck in my life? Would I still be alive today?

I know I would not be walking with the joy, hope, passion, and purpose that I live with today. I can say with confidence that I needed my ship to wreck in order for my path to change and true healing to come. Even if you are in the midst of a shipwreck in your life, I urge you to take courage and remember that your circumstances are equipping you to speak into the lives of others in a way that only you can.

God could have miraculously removed Paul from the situation on the ship, but He didn't. He allowed Paul to remain in his body, as a prisoner, still on a ship, and experience a shipwreck on top of that. We can get upset that God doesn't change our circumstances, but let's notice the beautiful way God encouraged Paul. He came to Paul in the midst of the trial and spoke encouragement to him. This story of Paul's miraculous courage in the face of trauma is indicative of the Christian life. The Holy Spirit gives the believer the power to say, "We are afflicted in every way but not crushed; we are perplexed but not in despair; we are persecuted but not abandoned; we are struck down but not destroyed" (2 Corinthians 4:8–9 CSB).

> When it was about daylight, Paul urged them all to take food, saying, "Today is the fourteenth day that you have been waiting and going without food, having eaten nothing. So I urge you to take some food. For this is for your survival, since none of you will lose a hair from your head." After he said these things and had taken some bread, he gave thanks to God in the presence of all of them, and after he broke it, he began to eat. They all were encouraged and took food themselves. In all there were 276 of us on the ship. When they had eaten enough, they began to lighten the ship by throwing the grain overboard into the sea. (Acts 27:33–38 CSB)

After two weeks of suffering, did you notice the state of Paul's heart? He was able to encourage the other passengers to nourish themselves. Sometimes the best thing you can do is get up and eat, or shower, or take your prescribed medication. There are tangible things in life that strengthen us to continue on the journey the Lord has us on. And, most notably, there was thankfulness flowing from him. He was able to give thanks to God in the presence of all the men. Thankfulness is a pathway to joy even in midst of the most harrowing experience.

The ship eventually wrecked, and like God revealed to Paul, everyone safely reached the shore. The rest of Acts tells the story of Paul in Rome. Paul was allowed to live by himself, but he was guarded by a soldier and considered under house arrest. "Paul stayed two whole years in his own rented house. And he welcomed all who visited him, proclaiming the kingdom of God and teaching about the Lord Jesus Christ with all boldness and without hindrance" (Acts 28:30–31 CSB). But he was a prisoner. How can a man under house arrest be called unhindered?

Unhindered.

Not slowed.

Not forbidden.

Not blocked.

Not interfered with.

Paul was hindered in various ways in his life, yet he trusted his life to the sovereign God, living like one who knew that everything happened was for his good and God's glory. Paul did not waste his time in prison. It was while he was arrested in that house in Rome that he penned letters to the Ephesians, Philippians, Colossians, and to Philemon. Out from a situation the human mind would deem absolutely hindered, flowed some of the most beautiful and encouraging scripture of all time.

To the Ephesians he wrote,

> I pray that out of his glorious riches he may strengthen you with power through his Spirit in your inner being, so that Christ may dwell in your hearts through faith. And I pray that you, being rooted and established in love, may have power, together with all the Lord's holy people, to grasp how wide and long and high and deep is the love of Christ, and to know this love that surpasses knowledge—that you may be filled to the measure of all the fullness of God. (Ephesians 3:16–19)

To the Philippians he wrote: "Now I want you to know, brothers and sisters, that what has happened to me has actually advanced the gospel, so that it has become known throughout the whole imperial guard, and to everyone else, that my imprisonment is because I am in Christ. Most of the brothers have gained confidence in the Lord from my imprisonment and dare even more to speak the word fearlessly" (Philippians 1:12–14 CSB).

To the Colossians he wrote:

> We are asking that you may be filled with the knowledge of his will in all wisdom and spiritual understanding, so that you may walk worthy of the Lord, fully pleasing to him: bearing fruit in every good work and growing in the knowledge of God, being strengthened with all power, according to his glorious might, so that you may have great endurance and patience, joyfully giving thanks to the Father, who has enabled you to share in the saints' inheritance in the light. He has rescued us from the domain of darkness and transferred us into the kingdom of the Son he loves.
> (Colossians 1:9–13 CSB)

To Philemon he wrote: "I always thank my God when I mention you in my prayers, because I hear of your love for all the saints and the faith that you have in the Lord Jesus. I pray that your participation in the faith may become effective through knowing every good thing that is in us for the glory of Christ" (Philemon 1:4–6 CSB).

The words Paul wrote long ago are still alive and active today, only proving that "the word of God is not bound" (2 Timothy 2:9 CSB). It is unstoppable. It cannot be blocked. It was not hindered then, and it never will be hindered. Paul was human. He wrestled with sin. He knew what it was like to have scars on his body from abuse, emotional pain that could resurface unannounced, and relationship strife that could awaken bitterness within his heart. But this man knew who he belonged to and was committed to serve the One who stood by him. He held fast to God's promises and his action flowed from a mind fully stayed on Him. He lived the very instruction he sent to the Colossians: "Set your minds on things above, not on earthly things" (Colossians 3:2). Setting our minds— even minds with mental illness—on things above redirects the earthly view of pain to the heavenly view of purpose.

Paul was a man of hope. Biblical hope doesn't just desire something good for the future, it expects it. Hope allows a perspective that sees purpose in pain, supernaturally unhindering the hindered believer. And even though Paul was bound, God's Word was not. Maybe it's an illness or trauma from the past that seemingly hinders your ministry today. But what if what you see as a hindrance is the very thing that sets you apart for your specific purpose? What if that "hindrance" is what draws others to your unhindered hope?

But how could mental illness ever set you apart for your specific purpose? Depression and PTSD, once they reared their ugly heads, led our family to relocate back home to Oklahoma. I was crushed. I went from a woman walking the streets of Turkey with absolute purpose to a woman in the Bible Belt who couldn't see her purpose at all.

Mental illness wrecked my limited view of how the Lord could ever use me. After a year of healing and thinking we would move back to Turkey, the most devastating opinion was spoken over me by a fellow believer, and I received it as absolute truth. I was told I was no longer suitable for ministry. It's as if there was a flaw in me that somehow hindered my ability to love others and share Jesus.

And guess what. I believed them.

Having embraced the identity of unsuitable, the confidence I once possessed in my capacity to be used by the Lord, vanished. It's as though they felt that the darkness of my struggle with depression overshadowed the new chapter of survival God wove into my story that was begging to be shared. It has taken a long time for the veil to lift from my eyes, but I can now see with God-given clarity. Mental illness does not cancel you from being useful in the kingdom of God, but rather increases the very ministry God has given you on this earth.

Depression has often left me feeling imprisoned in my body and mind. The fatigue and overwhelming feelings of sadness can chain me to darkness, interfering with my ministry from a human perspective. But what if we shifted our perspective? If God's power is made perfect in our weakness, then could depression be a gift? If joy is a fruit of the Spirit within believers, then could your overwhelming sadness set the stage for your Spirit-filled joy to shine with all the radiance of Christ?

What if we embraced our frail humanity that is likened to a clay jar in scripture, "For God, who said, 'Let light shine out of darkness,' made his light shine in our hearts to give us the light of the knowledge of God's glory displayed in the face of Christ. But we have this treasure in jars of clay to show that this all-surpassing power is from God and not from us" (2 Corinthians 4:6–7).

The intensity of mental illness can sometimes ebb and flow. On the days that depression cripples you from leaving your bed, simply choosing to live is glorifying God. When anxiety sends you spinning out of control, asking a friend for prayer or tangible help, shows the onlooking world the love of Christ within the Body. Being used by God in the midst of mental illness does not have to look like writing a book or speaking on a stage. There is beauty in the everyday moments where even your choice to simply endure is an act of faith, knowing that perseverance is worth it.

Charles Spurgeon, who suffered from deep depression, knew well what it was like to preach hope from a hindered place:

> One Sabbath morning, I preached from the text, "My God, My God, why has Thou forsaken Me?" and though I did not say so, yet I preached my own experience. I heard my own chains clank while I tried to preach to my fellow-prisoners in the dark; but I could not tell why I was brought into such an awful horror of darkness, for which I condemned myself.
>
> On the following Monday evening, a man came to see me who bore all the marks of despair upon his countenance. His hair seemed to stand up right, and his

eyes were ready to start from their sockets. He said to me, after a little parleying, "I never before, in my life, heard any man speak who seemed to know my heart. Mine is a terrible case; but on Sunday morning you painted me to the life and preached as if you had been inside my soul."

By God's grace I saved that man from suicide and led him into gospel light and liberty; but I know I could not have done it if I had not myself been confined in the dungeon in which he lay. I tell you the story, brethren, because you sometimes may not understand your own experience, and the perfect people may condemn you for having it; but what know they of God's servants? You and I have to suffer much for the sake of the people of our charge.

You may be in Egyptian darkness, and you may wonder why such a horror chills your marrow; but you may be altogether in the pursuit of your calling and be led of the Spirit to a position of sympathy with desponding minds.[4]

Broken people are not drawn to perfection, they are drawn to the broken person walking in wholeness through a relationship with Christ. No one can understand living with mental illness like one who lives with it. To the believer who loves Jesus but has felt disqualified from His work because of struggling, grief, trauma, or mental illness, God delights in displaying His power through our humanity.

Trials humanize us. The ones lost in darkness will undoubtedly see His Light shine through the cracks of broken minds that are captivated by Christ and securely held in the hands of the One who fashioned them. We all need God. Nothing has made me poorer in spirit, recognizing my need for God's help, like mental illness. According to Jesus, that makes me blessed, for "Blessed are the poor in spirit, for the kingdom of heaven is theirs" (Matthew 5:3 CSB). And that makes you blessed too.

11

Encouragement for the Loved Ones

I spent many hours on a couch of a friend. It was in the same spot every Thursday that I slowly emerged from the stronghold of shame that I didn't realize held me captive until she gently pointed it out. I received her words because she had proven by her consistent love and acceptance that she was a safe place. There was a spirit-filled and grace-laden connection between us.

Engulfed in shame, I couldn't see how it ruled my affections and thoughts, eventually producing allegiance to wrong and sinful actions. Shame kept my face turned from God. He didn't turn His face from me; it was my bowed down face and slumped shoulders that kept me from running into His embrace.

It was through consistent human connection that I gained courage to be vulnerable, even admitting that I doubted my salvation. Through my friend's safety, a reflection of Christ's, I started to see the danger of the fortress I was trapped in. God used a tangible human refuge to show me the perfect refuge that He is. My vulnerability with her led to vulnerability with Him. I was blind, but through the love of another, I began to see.

He is the shield that surrounds us and the One who lifts our heads. When we look to Him, our shame is replaced with radiance. A mentally ill Christian imprisoned in the stronghold of shame, where the belief "I am bad" becomes the notion through which all is seen, is more likely to entertain suicidal thoughts. A mentally ill Christian held safely in the stronghold of God, where the belief that "I am weak, but He is strong" becomes the mental antidote to the enemy's lies, is more likely to live in freedom and purpose even if suicidal thoughts continue to batter their mind.

There was a beautiful dance happening with my friend as she came in close and proved that she was in the fight with me. I, too, came in close and started to open up about the darkest struggles in my heart. Her presence became a safe haven where my belief that I was a burden would be challenged. I truly believed that my life was a burden on my loved ones. I felt guilty and therefore stayed silent about my struggles. But one day, as the Lord so faithfully does, He took me to the Word and showed me the beauty of bearing one another's burdens, and how this is what true community does for each other.

In the letter Paul wrote to the Galatians, he said: "Brothers and sisters, if someone is caught in a sin, you who live by the Spirit should restore that person gently. But watch yourselves, or you also may be tempted. Carry each other's burdens, and in this way you will fulfill the law of Christ" (Galatians 6:1–2). If you'll notice, "this brother was 'overtaken' in a fault. This is quite a different thing than OVERTAKING a sin. Some people go looking for sin, and go out of their way to find it. But this is not the case in our Scripture. This brother was 'overtaken,' implying that he was trying to get away from it, trying to avoid it, but because of weakness, failure of prayer, or failure to look to the Lord for victory, was overtaken. It was not deliberate sinning, but being 'overcome' in a moment of weakness."[1]

Mental illness, which is not in and of itself a sin, unfortunately becomes the perfect atmosphere for a surprise attack, or rather a surprise intrusive thought, that suggests hard to resist sin when the mind is in need of help. When all is dark and you yearn for it to stop, surprise suggestions of ways to numb the pain not only become worthy of notice, they become enticing.

While reading Galatians, it became startlingly clear that my friend's invitation into her life with the freedom to be myself was her obeying Jesus. Her bearing my burdens was her obeying Christ when he taught His disciples to love the Lord with all their hearts and to love others as they would love themselves.

If I were to hide from the friend the Lord graciously provided to walk alongside me in the battle, I would be hindering her from obeying Christ, which is where true joy is found. When the label of "burden" would attempt to silence me, the Holy Spirit would remind me that it was biblical what she was doing when she carried my burdens with me. It was OK to let her bear my burdens, and the more I did, with Jesus always remaining my Savior, the more comfortable I became confessing to her the sins that I was struggling with and asking God for forgiveness from a true, repentant heart.

When I confessed the sin that dominated me, she would restore me by speaking truth of Scripture to me, loving me in spite of my failure, and praying with and for me. The word "restore" in Galatians 6:1 has the idea of mending that which is broken, or of setting a bone that has been dislocated. If your loved one falls down and breaks their leg, would you leave them there to suffer alone, or would you give them a hand and help them? This is the idea here; this is a beautiful picture of loving the Lord and loving others.

To allow loved ones to carry my burdens alongside me, took humility, vulnerability and saying no to the enemy's scheme of shame, always remembering that "now there is no condemnation for those who belong to Christ Jesus" (Romans 8:1 NLT). No longer was staying silent and fighting alone an option. Like James writes in James 5:16 (AMPC), "Confess to one another therefore your faults (your slips, your false steps, your offenses, your sins) and pray [also] for one another, that you may be healed and restored [to a spiritual tone of mind and heart]. The earnest (heartfelt, continued) prayer of a righteous man makes tremendous power available [dynamic in its working]."

We are commanded in Scripture to confess our sins to one another and pray for each other. Do we need others to find forgiveness in Christ? No, for salvation comes through Christ alone. But are we meant to just flounder alone in the battle against sin and the enemy? No, we are meant to do life together, and the more I embraced a lifestyle of accountability, the more joy I found in actually being known and seen—not judged and reprimanded—but loved, cared for, listened to, and prayed over.

Struggle like Epaphras

My friend's struggle in prayer on my behalf is no new thing, for even in Scripture we see a man named Epaphras who intentionally wrestled in prayer on the behalf of others. Epaphras was also very likely both the planter and pastor of the Colossian church. "The church of Colossae apparently got its start during Paul's three-year ministry in Ephesus. During this time, a Colossians named Epaphras probably traveled to Ephesus and responded to Paul's proclamation of the gospel" (Acts 19:10).

"The new believer returned to his hometown and began sharing the good news of Christ, which resulted in the birth of the Colossian church (Col. 1:7)."[2] In Colossians 1:7 (CSB), Paul calls Epaphras a "dearly loved fellow servant," also saying that "He is a faithful minister of Christ." Paul states in his letter to the Colossians that "Epaphras, who is one of you, a servant of Christ Jesus, greets you, always struggling on your behalf in his prayers, that you may stand mature and fully assured in all the will of God" (Colossians 4:12 ESV). Other versions of the Bible describe him this way: "Epaphras, who is one of you and a bond-servant of Christ Jesus, sends you greetings. [He is] always striving for you in his prayers, praying with genuine concern, [pleading] that you may [as people of character and courage] stand firm, [spiritually mature] and fully assured in all the will of God" (AMP), and "Epaphras, who is one of you, a servant of Christ Jesus, sends you greetings. He is always wrestling for you in his prayers. so that you can stand mature and fully assured in everything God wills" (CSB).

The way Epaphras loved and faithfully prayed for the Colossians, as well as other Christians in nearby cities, is a beautiful example for us today. He was always striving, struggling, laboring, and pleading on the behalf of others. This is the dedication I felt from the prayers I heard prayed over me from my friend as I would hold her hand and hear her go to God on my behalf. This is the dedication I noticed when other friends would repeatedly message me prayers and verses they were speaking over me. As found in 1 Thessalonians 5:14 (ESV), I "urge you, brothers, admonish the idle, encourage the fainthearted, help the weak, be patient with them all."

Maybe you love someone who struggles with mental illness, and you have grown weary in believing your prayers matter. They absolutely do, and when we look at the intensity in which Epaphras struggled in prayer for Christians, we can see that the struggle you feel in praying is not only normal but modeled for us in Scripture. In Greek, the word struggle (*agōnízomai*) means conflict. It also means "To contend for victory in the public games (1 Cor. 9:25). It generally came to mean to fight, wrestle (John 18:36). Figuratively, it is the task of faith in persevering amid temptation and opposition

(1 Tim. 6:12; 2 Tim. 4:7). It also came to mean to take pains, to wrestle as in an award contest, straining every nerve to the uttermost toward the goal (Luke 13:24 [cf. 1 Cor. 9:25; Phil. 3:12ff.; Heb. 4:1])."[3]

To the one struggling, ask God to give you the courage to be transparent with a loved one, for in vulnerability and humility, we find freedom and strength.

To the one who loves a struggling one, ask God to give you the ability to faithfully struggle in prayer on their behalf. Your prayers matter. Hearing you pray over them will undoubtedly strengthen their hope, and seeing your prayers answered will convince them that they are not alone in the battle.

Pray for your struggling loved ones. Let them hear your prayers on their behalf. I am a living testimony to the power of prayer and how the word "impossible" is erased when we take requests to the living God. My friend has not fixed me, and has even admitted to feeling helpless in the struggle, but I can say with confidence that her prayers have mattered and helped me hold on some days that I thought depression really might be the death of me.

If you are the loved one of someone struggling with mental illness, I know you must go through moments of feeling helpless, but remember that in your helplessness you have been given the Helper. Jesus said, "But the Helper, the Holy Spirit, whom the Father will send in my name, he will teach you all things and bring to your remembrance all that I have said to you. Peace I leave with you; my peace I give to you. Not as the world gives do I give to you. Let not your hearts be troubled, neither let them be afraid" (John 14:26–27 ESV). May you love through the strength and wisdom the Helper provides and walk in peace as you keep your eyes bravely locked on Jesus.

Epilogue

The Ultimate Example
of Joyful Sorrow

One of the greatest examples of what I call "joyful sorrow" is the Easter story. For the followers of Jesus, Friday was traumatic, and Sunday was joyful, but Saturday was just Saturday. Saturday was silence, broken dreams, questions, grief, and reeling from the trauma of witnessing the graphic murder of Jesus. Saturday is the day that rests in the tension of death and life; of brokenness and healing; of sorrow and joy. This is the day that silence and waiting become developers of faith and hope. Without waiting how could we learn trust? If our eyes could see all God is doing, how could we learn to see the unseen? Without circumstances seeming hopeless, how could we learn to exercise the remarkable gift of expectant hope that Jesus has given us?

Sometimes life can feel like a continual Saturday where God seems quiet. Saturday can feel like the enemy's favorite day to torment, but the silence of Saturday is often where faith is forged and mountains are moved.

As the Lord allows us to wait, trusting in His promises opens our eyes of faith, directing them forward as we wait for

Sunday. Weeping may tarry for the night, but joy comes with morning. Mental illness may persist in your body, but someday things will all be made right, for "He will wipe away every tear from their eyes. Death will be no more; grief, crying, and pain will be no more, because the previous things have passed away" (Revelation 21:4 CSB). Saturday was only temporary and while Jesus remained dead, God's plan of redemption was in the process of making beauty from ashes, and His plan of redemption in our life is also in motion.

Jesus knew God would not forsake Him to that grave and we need to believe this as well. Silence does not equal abandonment or inactivity. God is always working and Sunday is always coming.

God could rescue us immediately from every situation, or even just prevent it from happening, but there is so much we'd miss out on. The Bible is full of waiting moments. Before the sea was parted; before the dead were raised; before eyesight restored; before lion mouths were shut; before prisoners released; before the miracle, came the wait. We could be spared the painful sorrow of the circumstance, but nothing compares to the joy of witnessing God in all His power, glory, and strength as He comes through in His perfect way. The coming resurrection is worth enduring the death.

If you are in this continual state of "Saturday," remember that it is so very special and full of purpose. Yes, the past may have been traumatic and today may be a day of waiting and sorrow, but God is working.

His joy sustains, His hope gives courage, and Sunday will be here soon.

A Final Word

When I finished this book of hope that God whispered to my heart long ago, I sat on my porch in small town Oklahoma, contemplating the simple suicide note of despair I penned several months prior. I am amazed at the miracle of not only being alive today, but that He would bring this vision to fruition. It has not been easy to share my story and the intimate lessons the Lord taught me as I fought hard for life, but as I sit here wrapping up what has been not only a labor of love, but an act of worship to my Father, I can say with confidence that it has all been worth it.

You are worth it.

And now it's your turn. I have been praying while writing that you will have encountered Jesus through these pages and the Scripture referenced, and that your hope would burn bright with expectation for all that He has for you.

May you walk with purpose in your suffering, remembering that God is with you and will never abandon you. Your story matters and is meant to be told. Remember, your voice may tremble as you share your testimony, but so will the demons.

I hope with all of my heart that as you begin sharing with others how the Lord sustains you in your weakness, that you will experience the miraculous joy that really can be yours even in your sorrow, for "Consider it a great joy, my brothers and sisters, whenever you experience various trials, because you know that the testing of your faith produces endurance. And let endurance have its full effect, so that you may be mature and complete, lacking nothing" (James 1:2–4 CSB).

In parting, I want to share one last verse with you that I pray you will never forget in a moment of weakness:

> Therefore do not let sin reign in your mortal body so that you obey its evil desires. Do not offer any part of yourself to sin as an instrument of wickedness, but rather offer yourselves to God as those who have been brought from death to life; and offer every part of yourself to him as an instrument of righteousness. For sin shall no longer be your master, because you are not under the law, but under grace. (Romans 6:12–14)

You, fellow believer who struggles, and may even desire to die, live in the tension of what God has already done and the responsibility that rests on you as His child. You may still be tempted by sinful desires, but you must live with the resolve to not let those desires to sin control you. Each day, when you wake up to His new mercies, give yourself afresh to your King. God has conquered you so sin doesn't have to. Remember that you are no longer a slave to sin, for you are free. Your mortal body may desire to surrender to the pain, but you were made for perseverance, joy, victory, and the abundant life even when your mind struggles.

You are more than a conqueror who can have joy even in sorrow.

Thank you, Jesus, to You be all the glory, amen.

Notes

1. Healing Starts with Humility

1. American Psychiatric Association, *Diagnostic and Statistical Manual of Mental Disorders*, Fifth Edition (American Psychiatric Association, 2013), 176. Hereafter referred to as DSM-5.
2. DSM-5, 142.
3. DSM-5, 164.
4. "What Is Electroconvulsive Therapy (ECT)," Psychiatry.org, July 2019, www.psychiatry.org/patients-families/ect.

2. Feasting in the Valley

1. Bessel A. van der Kolk, *The Body Keeps the Score: Brain, Mind, and Body in the Healing of Trauma* (New York: Penguin, 2014), 3.
2. Elizabeth Wurtzel, *Prozac Nation: Young and Depressed in America* (New York: Riverhead, 1995), 191.
3. Elisabeth Elliot, *Finding Your Way Through Loneliness* (Grand Rapids: Revell, 2001), 27.
4. Curt Thompson, *The Soul of Shame: Retelling the Stories We Believe About Ourselves* (Downers Grove, IL: InterVarsity Press, 2105), 29.
5. Thompson, *Soul of Shame*, 31.
6. Thompson, *Soul of Shame*, 124.
7. Susan Hunt, *Spiritual Mothering: The Titus 2 Model for Women Mentoring Women* (Wheaton, IL: Crossway, 1992), 125.
8. Hunt, *Spiritual Mothering*, 150.
9. Hunt, *Spiritual Mothering*, 150.

10. van der Kolk, *Body Keeps the Score*, 212.
11. van der Kolk, *Body Keeps the Score*, 212.

3. A Thorn in My Mind

1. Dorothy Kelley Patterson and Rhonda Harrington Kelley, eds., *Women's Evangelical Commentary: New Testament* (Nashville: Holman, 2006), 502–3.
2. C. H. Spurgeon, "The Thorn in the Flesh" (sermon, Metropolitan Tabernacle, Newington, December 8, 1872), 5; www.spurgeon gems.org/sermon/chs1084.pdf.
3. Spiros Zodhiates, *The Complete Word Study Dictionary: New Testament* (Chattanooga, TN: AMG Publishers, 2002), electronic edition.
4. Zodhiates, *Complete Word Study Dictionary*.
5. Patterson and Kelley, *Women's Evangelical Commentary*, 503–4.

4. Sober-Minded

1. DSM-5, 164.
2. Dorothy Kelley Patterson and Rhonda Harrington Kelley, eds., *Women's Evangelical Commentary: New Testament* (Nashville: Holman, 2006), 797.
3. Patterson and Kelley, *Women's Evangelical Commentary*.
4. Patterson and Kelley, *Women's Evangelical Commentary*.
5. ESV Study Bible (Wheaton, IL: Crossway, 2008), James 1:15.
6. "1 Thessalonians 5:8 Commentary," Precept Austin, April 28, 2020, www.preceptaustin.org/1thessalonians_58.
7. "1 Thessalonians 5:8," Precept Austin.
8. Sharon Jaynes, "Breaking Free of Strongholds and Strangleholds," Crosswalk.com, March 9, 2016, www.crosswalk.com/devotion als/girlfriends/breaking-free-of-strongholds-and-strangleholds -girlfriends-in-god-march-9-2016.html.
9. Steve Berger, "Winning the Mind Wars: Part 10—Anger and Loser Strongholds," Grace Chapel, March 24, 2013, https:// gracechapel.net/content/uploads/2017/10/Outline-20130324 .pdf.

10. "Colossians 3:2 Commentary," Precept Austin, February 2, 2020, https://www.preceptaustin.org/colossians_32.

11. ESV Study Bible, 2275.

12. William Barclay, *Barclay's Daily Study Bible Commentary: New Testament*, online at www.studylight.org/commentaries/eng/dsb .html.

13. Spiros Zodhiates, *The Complete Word Study Dictionary: New Testament* (Chattanooga, TN: AMG Publishers, 2002), electronic edition.

14. Barclay, *Barclay's Daily Study Bible Commentary*, Philippians 4.

15. Zodhiates, *Complete Word Study Dictionary*.

16. Stuart K. Weber, *Matthew*, Holman New Testament Commentary, ed. Max Anders (Nashville: Broadman & Holman, 2000), 40.

5. A Bound Daughter

1. ESV Study Bible (Wheaton, IL: Crossway, 2008), introduction to Luke.

2. ESV study Bible, introduction to Luke.

3. Spiros Zodhiates, *The Complete Word Study Dictionary: New Testament* (Chattanooga, TN: AMG Publishers, 2002), electronic edition.

4. Dorothy Kelley Patterson and Rhonda Harrington Kelley, eds., *Women's Evangelical Commentary: New Testament* (Nashville: Holman, 2006), 171.

5. Herbert Lockyer, *All the Miracles of the Bible* (Grand Rapids: Zondervan, 1961), 223.

6. Charles Haddon Spurgeon, "The Lifting Up of the Bowed Down" (sermon, Metropolitan Tabernacle, Newington, July 14, 1878), https://www.spurgeon.org/resource-library/sermons/the -lifting-up-of-the-bowed-down/#flipbook/.

7. ESV Study Bible, Luke 13:14.

8. Patterson and Kelley, *Women's Evangelical Commentary*, 224.

6. Mentally Ill for God's Glory

1. "2 Peter 1:6-7 Commentary," Precept Austin, April 26, 2021, www.preceptaustin.org/2_peter_16-7.

2. Oswald Chambers, *My Utmost for His Highest* (Grand Rapids: Discovery House, 1963), February 14.

3. Matthew Henry, *Matthew Henry's Concise Commentary on the Whole Bible* (Nashville: Thomas Nelson, 1997), 999.

4. "Barnes' Notes on the Bible," John 11:4, Bible Hub, https://biblehub.com/commentaries/john/11-4.htm.

5. Robert Jamieson, A. R. Fausset, and David Brown, *Commentary Critical and Explanatory on the Whole Bible*, Volume 2 (Oak Harbor, WA: Logos Research Systems, 1997), 148–49.

6. Dorothy Kelley Patterson and Rhonda Harrington Kelley, eds., *Women's Evangelical Commentary: New Testament* (Nashville: Holman, 2006), 227–28.

7. ESV Study Bible (Wheaton, IL: Crossway, 2008), John 11:25.

8. ESV Study Bible, John 11:35.

7. Watch and Pray

1. Dorothy Kelley Patterson and Rhonda Harrington Kelley, eds., *Women's Evangelical Commentary: New Testament* (Nashville: Holman, 2006), 355.

2. Patterson and Kelley, *Women's Evangelical Commentary*.

3. ESV Study Bible (Wheaton, IL: Crossway, 2008), Romans 6:6.

4. William Hendriksen and Simon J. Kistemaker, *Romans: Chapters 1–8*, New Testament Commentary (Grand Rapids: Baker Book House, 1980).

5. ESV Study Bible, Romans 6:12–13.

6. Patterson and Kelley, *Women's Evangelical Commentary*, 377.

7. "Romans 6:11 Commentary," Precept Austin, www.precept austin.org/romans_611-23.

8. ESV Study Bible, Romans 6:16.

9. Reza Negarestani, "The Corpse Bride: Thinking with *Nigredo*," www.thing.net/~rdom/ucsd/Zombies/The%20Corpse%20Bride.pdf, page 131; citing Jacques Brunschwig, "*Aristote et les pirates tyrrhéniens*," 1963.

10. Spiros Zodhiates, *The Complete Word Study Dictionary: New Testament* (Chattanooga, TN: AMG Publishers, 2002), electronic edition.

11. ESV Study Bible, 1832.
12. Zodhiates, *Complete Word Study Dictionary*.
13. Patterson and Kelley, *Women's Evangelical Commentary*, 765.
14. Patterson and Kelley, *Women's Evangelical Commentary*, 777.
15. Patterson and Kelley, *Women's Evangelical Commentary*, 777.
16. C. H. Spurgeon, "The Two Guards, Praying and Watching" (sermon, Metropolitan Tabernacle, Newington, May 1, 1892), 1; https://www.spurgeongems.org/sermon/chs2254.pdf.

9. Abiding with Mental Illness

1. ESV Study Bible (Wheaton, IL: Crossway, 2008), John 15:1–17.
2. Warren W. Wiersbe, *The Bible Exposition Commentary*, Vol. 1 (Wheaton, IL: Victor Books, 1996), 354–55.
3. John F. Walvoord and Roy B. Zuck, eds., *The Bible Knowledge Commentary: An Exposition of the Scriptures*, Vol. 2 (Wheaton, IL: Victor Books, 1985), 325.
4. Wiersbe, *Bible Exposition Commentary*, Vol. 1, 356.

10. Unhindered Hope

1. C. H. Spurgeon, "How to Become Fishers of Men" (sermon, Metropolitan Tabernacle, Newington, n.d.), 5.
2. Bessel A. van der Kolk, *The Body Keeps the Score: Brain, Mind, and Body in the Healing of Trauma* (New York: Penguin, 2014), 21.
3. van der Kolk, *Body Keeps the Score*, 30.
4. C. H. Spurgeon, *An All-Round Ministry: Addresses to Ministers and Students* (2017), 221–22.

11. Encouragement for the Loved Ones

1. "Galatians 6 Commentary," Precept Austin, January 7, 2022, www.preceptaustin.org/galatians-6-commentary.
2. ESV Study Bible (Wheaton, IL: Crossway, 2008), introduction to Colossians.
3. Spiros Zodhiates, *The Complete Word Study Dictionary: New Testament* (Chattanooga, TN: AMG Publishers, 2002), electronic edition.